Large Print Color B
Dachshunds
Adult Coloring Book

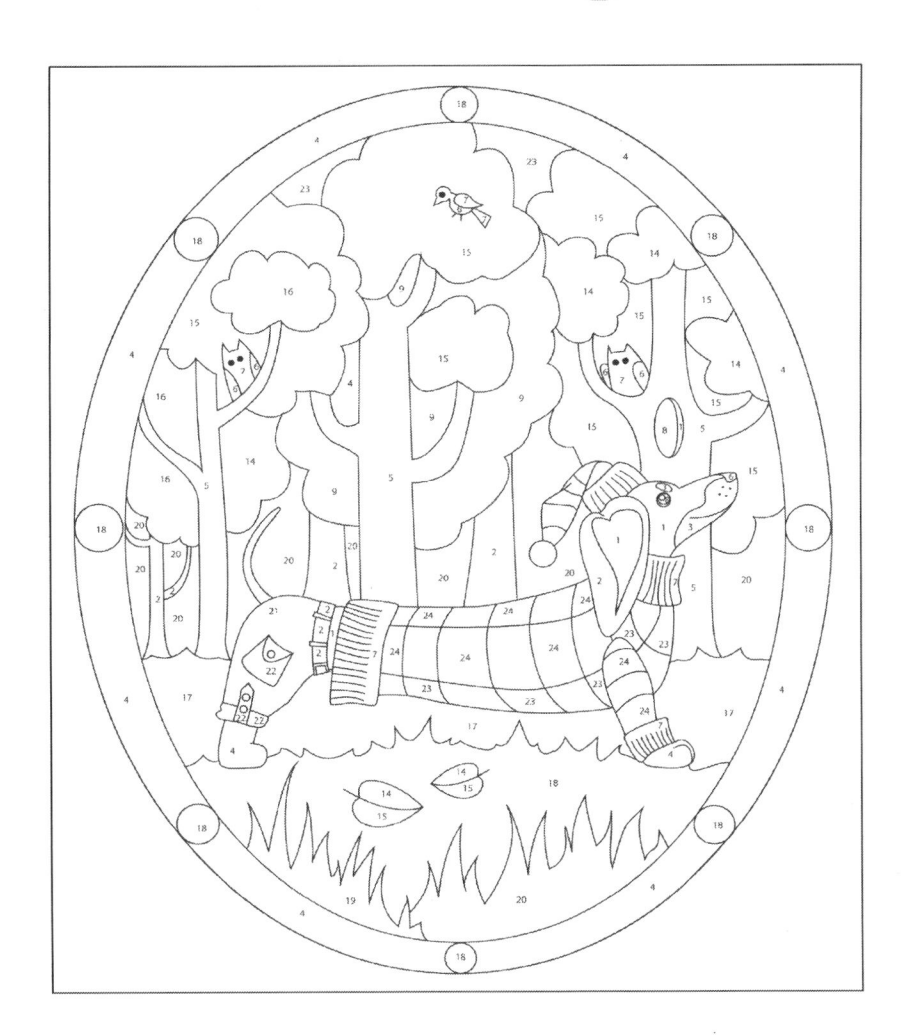

ZenMaster Coloring Books

Copyright © 2017 by ZenMaster
All rights reserved. No part of this publication may be reproduced, distributed, or transmitted in any form or by any means, including photocopying, recording, or other electronic or mechanical methods, without the prior written permission of the publisher.

Helpful Tips for Coloring

~ Sometimes the colors appear differently on paper than what you would expect. Use the color test page to play with your colors beforehand.

~ If you are using colored pencils make sure to keep them sharp. This helps when coloring smaller areas or details on the page. Fine point sharpies also work great for smaller areas.

~ Speaking of sharpies, make sure you put a scrap piece of paper behind the page you are coloring to keep the markers from bleeding to the next page.

~ When using crayons or pencils start out light. You can always go back and darken later.

~ There are so many tools for coloring: markers, sharpies, crayons, pencils, pastels, and the list goes on. Experiment with what works best for you and your designs. Though it's not necessary, using higher quality coloring utensils makes a difference.

~ If you come to a design that seems overwhelming just pick a place to start and go from there. Once you begin your creativity will quickly take over!! If you get discouraged just take a break and come back to the page later.

~ Remember to practice. Like anything else, the more you do it the better you'll get. It'll become more and more relaxing each time.

~ DON'T FOLLOW THE RULES! It's up to you how you color your designs. Just let your creativity take the lead and HAVE FUN!

COLOR TEST PAGE

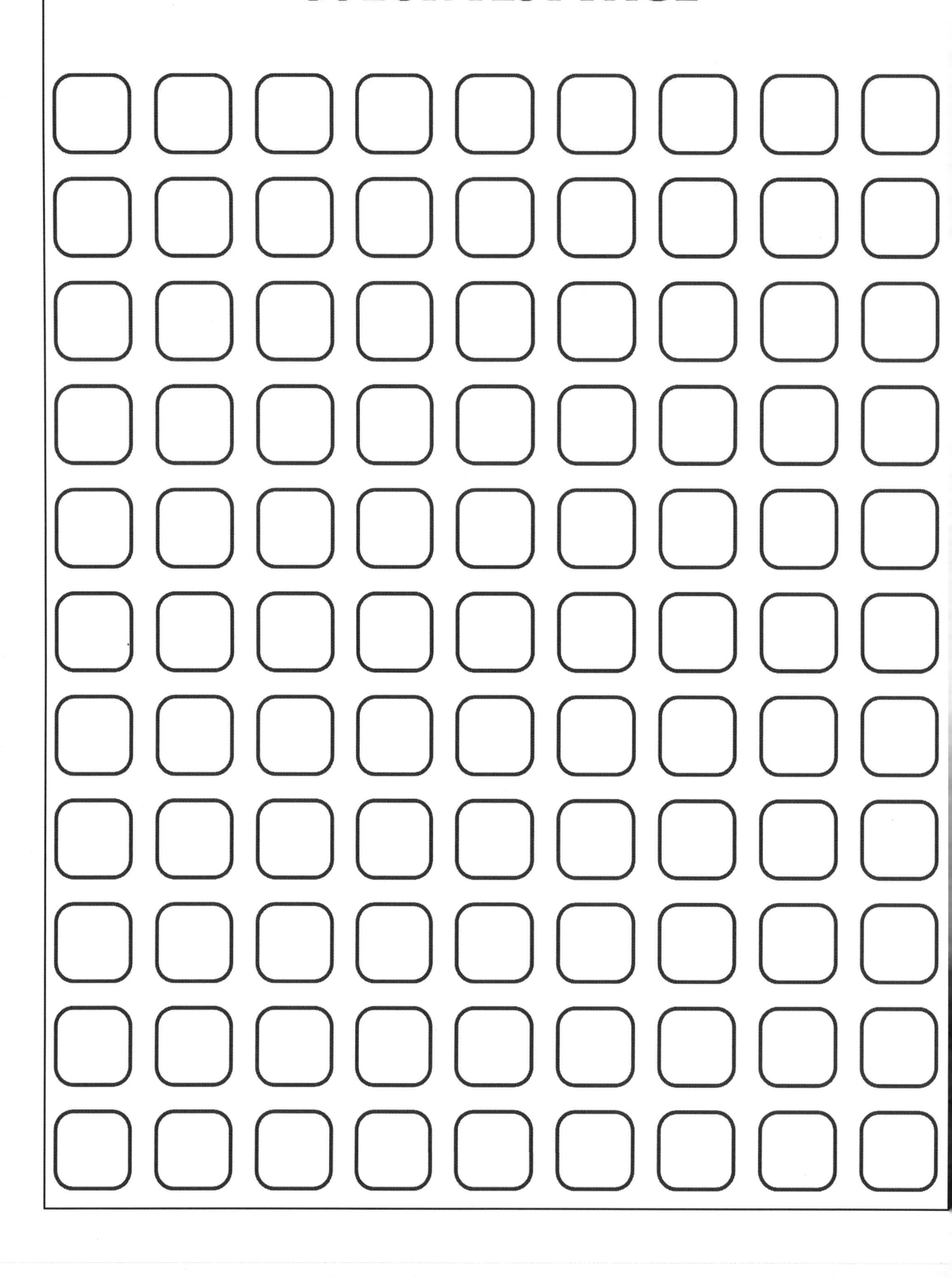

COLOR TEST PAGE

1. Dark Brown
2. Brown
3. Light Brown
4. Sand
5. Khaki
6. Dark Grey
7. Light Grey
8. Black
9. Light Pink
10. Pink
11. Magenta
12. Purple
13. Yellow
14. Gold
15. Orange
16. Red
17. Lime
18. Green
19. Light Green
20. Forrest Green
21. Blue Purple
22. Deep Blue
23. Sky Blue
24. Pale Blue

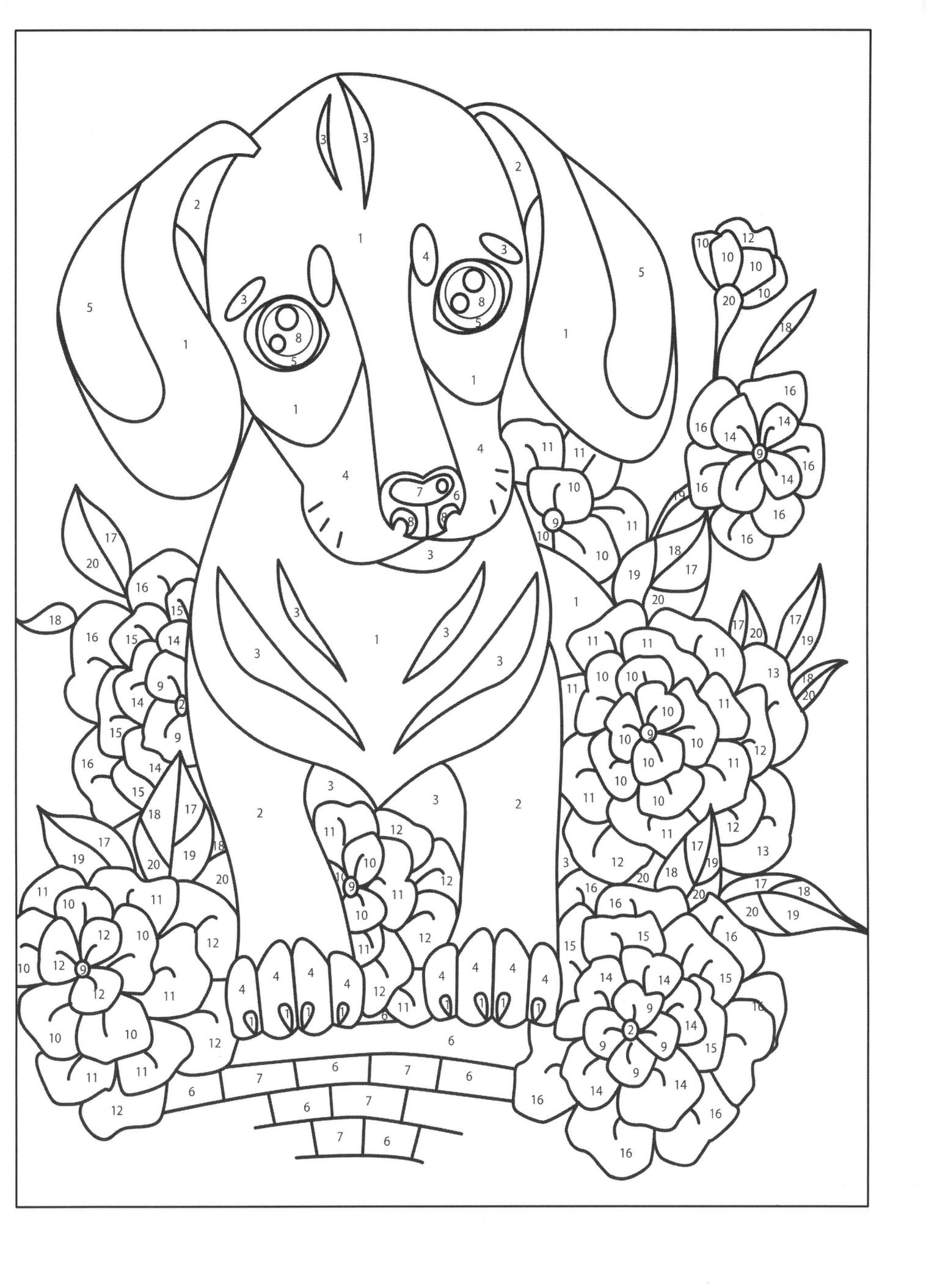

1. Dark Brown
2. Brown
3. Light Brown
4. Sand
5. Khaki
6. Dark Grey
7. Light Grey
8. Black
9. Light Pink
10. Pink
11. Magenta
12. Purple
13. Yellow
14. Gold
15. Orange
16. Red
17. Lime
18. Green
19. Light Green
20. Forrest Green
21. Blue Purple
22. Deep Blue
23. Sky Blue
24. Pale Blue

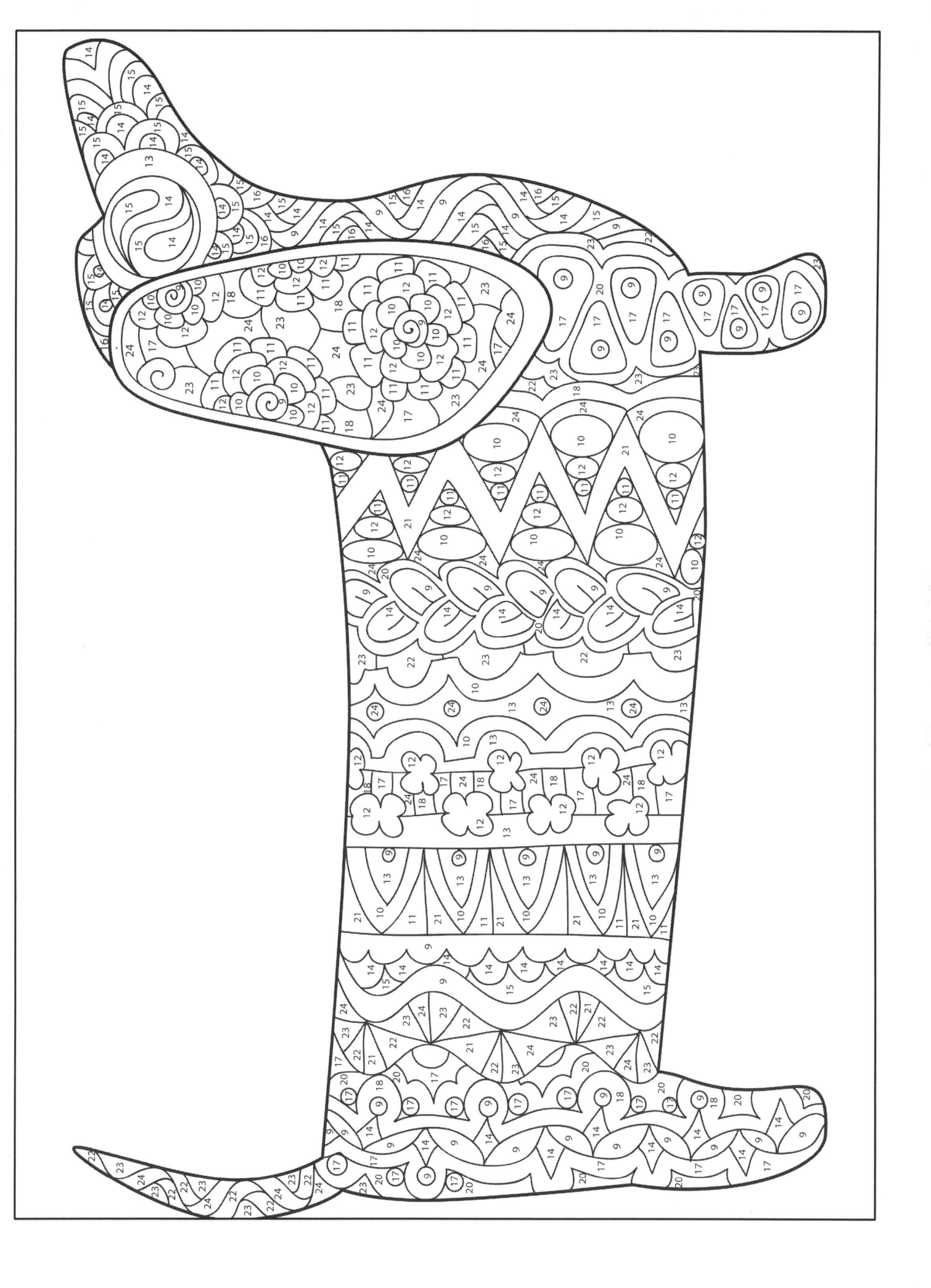

1. Dark Brown
2. Brown
3. Light Brown
4. Sand
5. Khaki
6. Dark Grey
7. Light Grey
8. Black
9. Light Pink
10. Pink
11. Magenta
12. Purple
13. Yellow
14. Gold
15. Orange
16. Red
17. Lime
18. Green
19. Light Green
20. Forrest Green
21. Blue Purple
22. Deep Blue
23. Sky Blue
24. Pale Blue

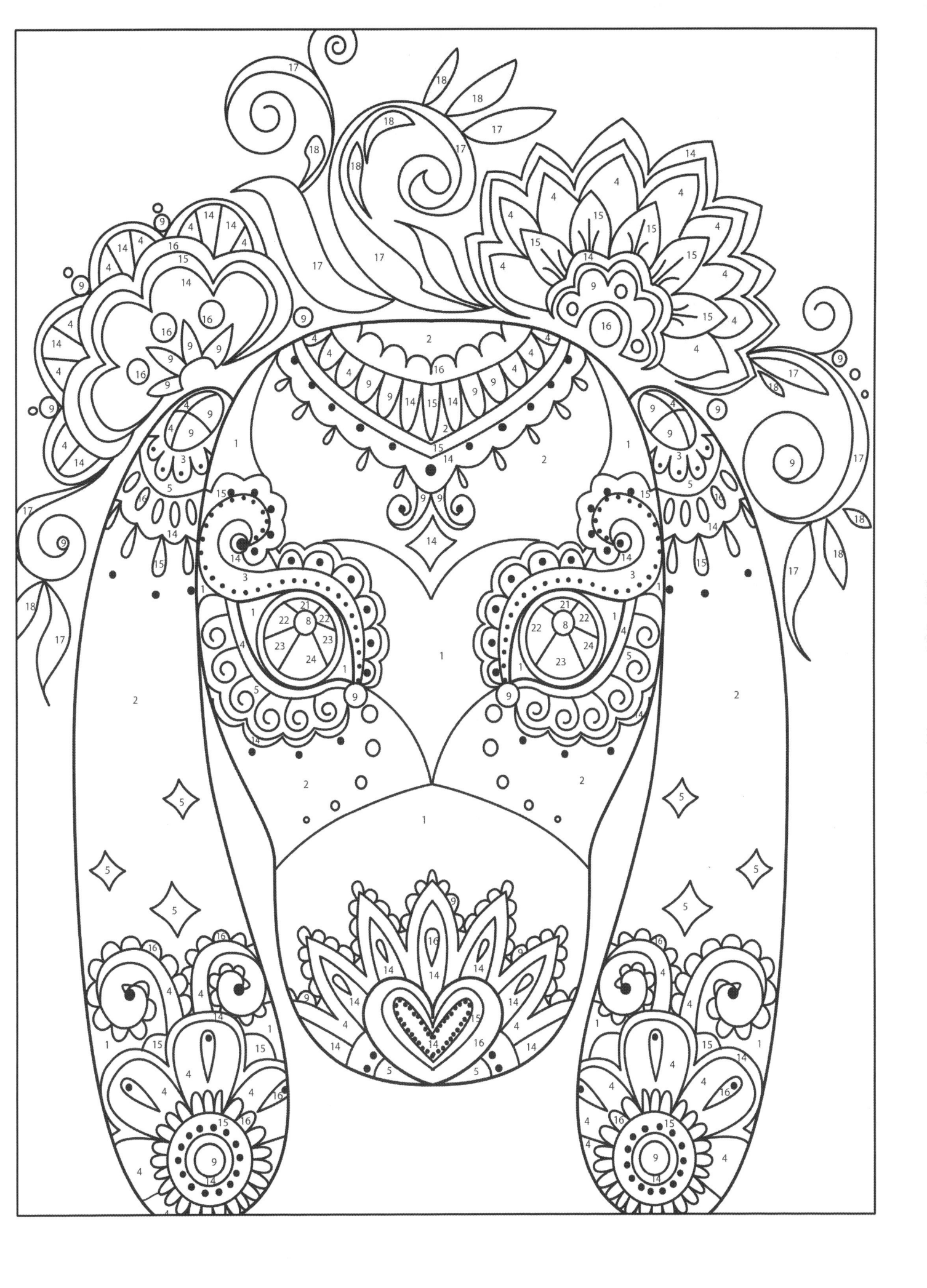

1. Dark Brown
2. Brown
3. Light Brown
4. Sand
5. Khaki
6. Dark Grey
7. Light Grey
8. Black
9. Light Pink
10. Pink
11. Magenta
12. Purple
13. Yellow
14. Gold
15. Orange
16. Red
17. Lime
18. Green
19. Light Green
20. Forrest Green
21. Blue Purple
22. Deep Blue
23. Sky Blue
24. Pale Blue

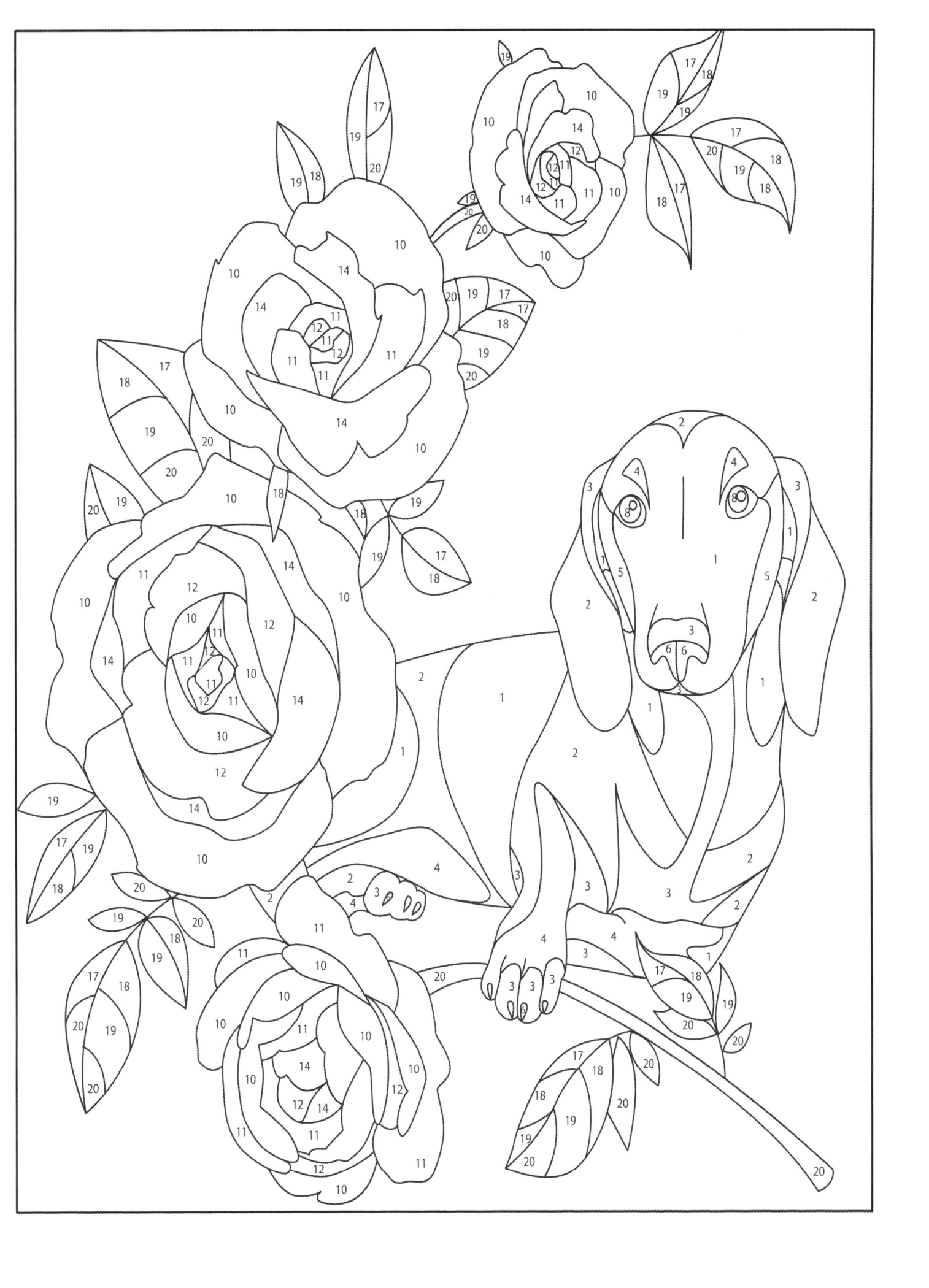

1. Dark Brown
2. Brown
3. Light Brown
4. Sand
5. Khaki
6. Dark Grey
7. Light Grey
8. Black
9. Light Pink
10. Pink
11. Magenta
12. Purple
13. Yellow
14. Gold
15. Orange
16. Red
17. Lime
18. Green
19. Light Green
20. Forrest Green
21. Blue Purple
22. Deep Blue
23. Sky Blue
24. Pale Blue

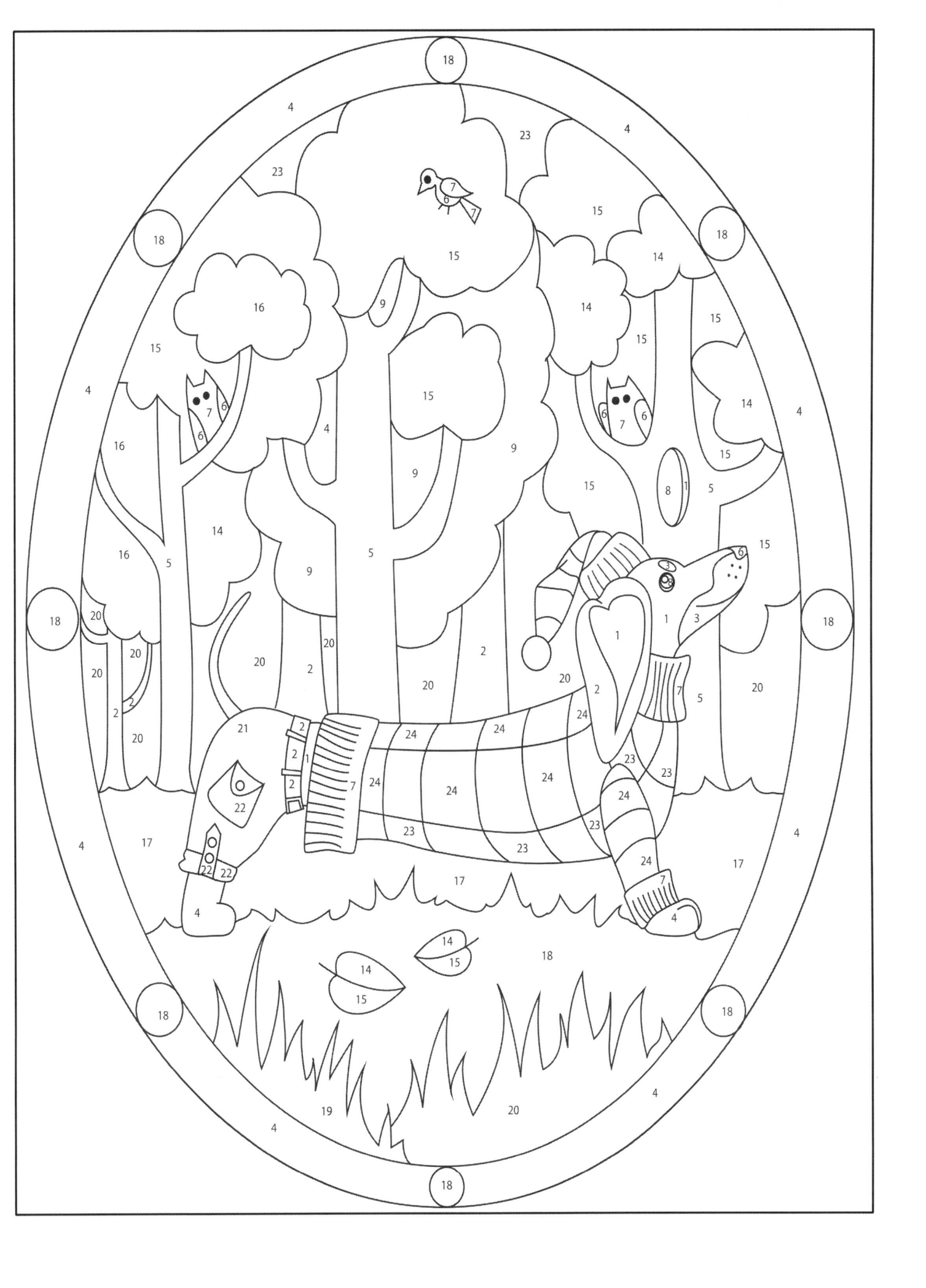

1. Dark Brown
2. Brown
3. Light Brown
4. Sand
5. Khaki
6. Dark Grey
7. Light Grey
8. Black
9. Light Pink
10. Pink
11. Magenta
12. Purple
13. Yellow
14. Gold
15. Orange
16. Red
17. Lime
18. Green
19. Light Green
20. Forrest Green
21. Blue Purple
22. Deep Blue
23. Sky Blue
24. Pale Blue

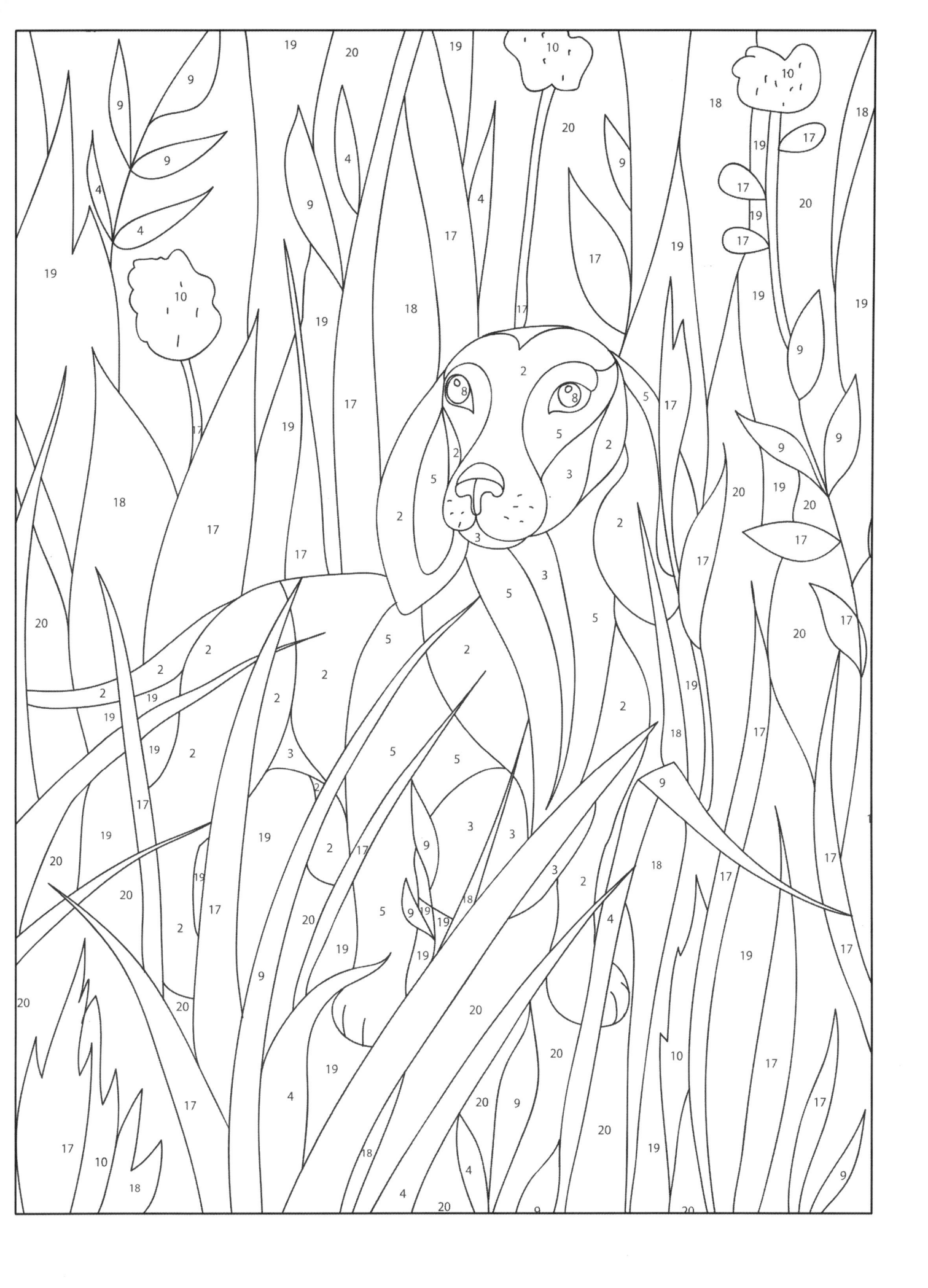

1. Dark Brown
2. Brown
3. Light Brown
4. Sand
5. Khaki
6. Dark Grey
7. Light Grey
8. Black
9. Light Pink
10. Pink
11. Magenta
12. Purple
13. Yellow
14. Gold
15. Orange
16. Red
17. Lime
18. Green
19. Light Green
20. Forrest Green
21. Blue Purple
22. Deep Blue
23. Sky Blue
24. Pale Blue

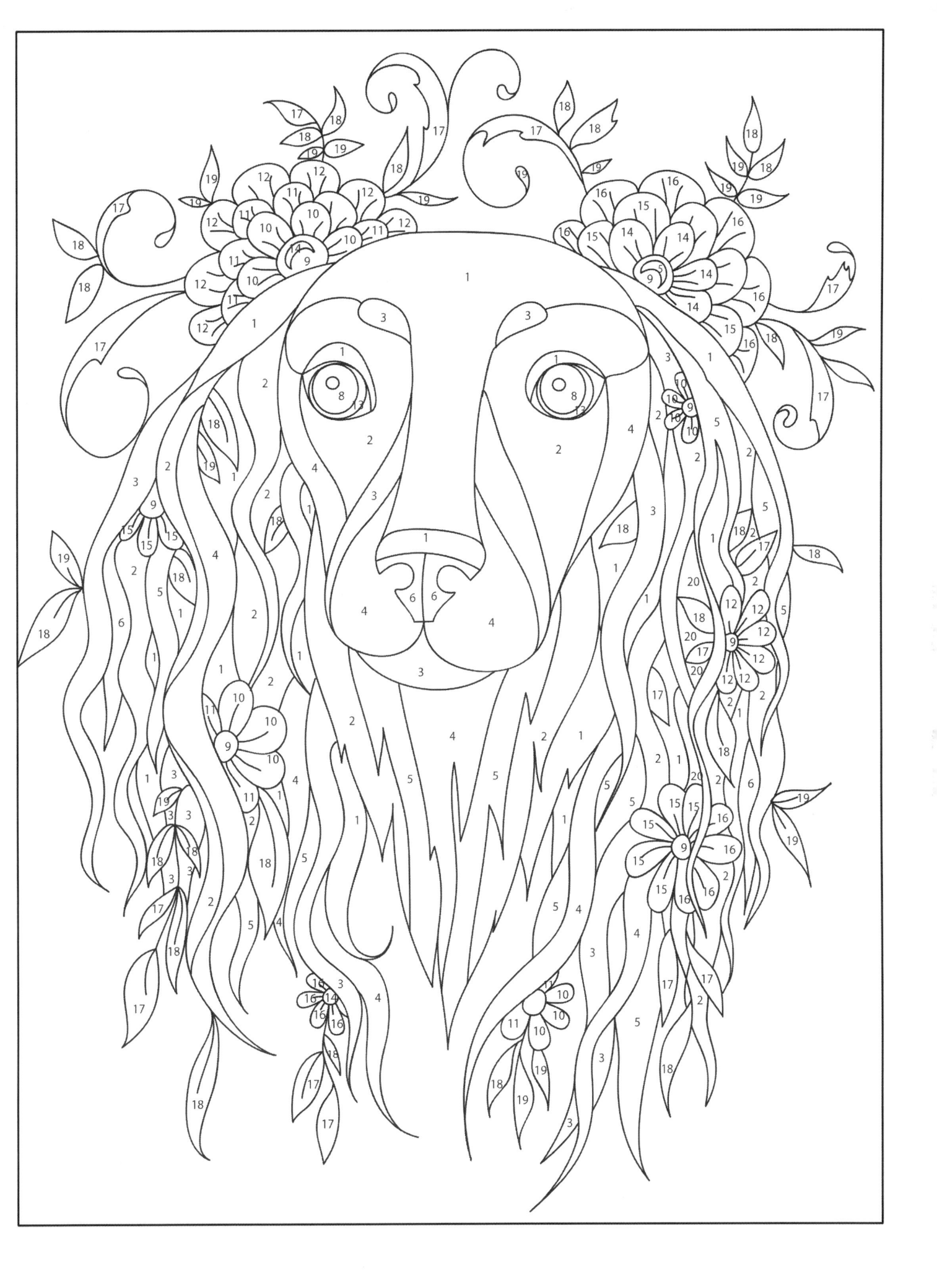

1. Dark Brown
2. Brown
3. Light Brown
4. Sand
5. Khaki
6. Dark Grey
7. Light Grey
8. Black
9. Light Pink
10. Pink
11. Magenta
12. Purple
13. Yellow
14. Gold
15. Orange
16. Red
17. Lime
18. Green
19. Light Green
20. Forrest Green
21. Blue Purple
22. Deep Blue
23. Sky Blue
24. Pale Blue

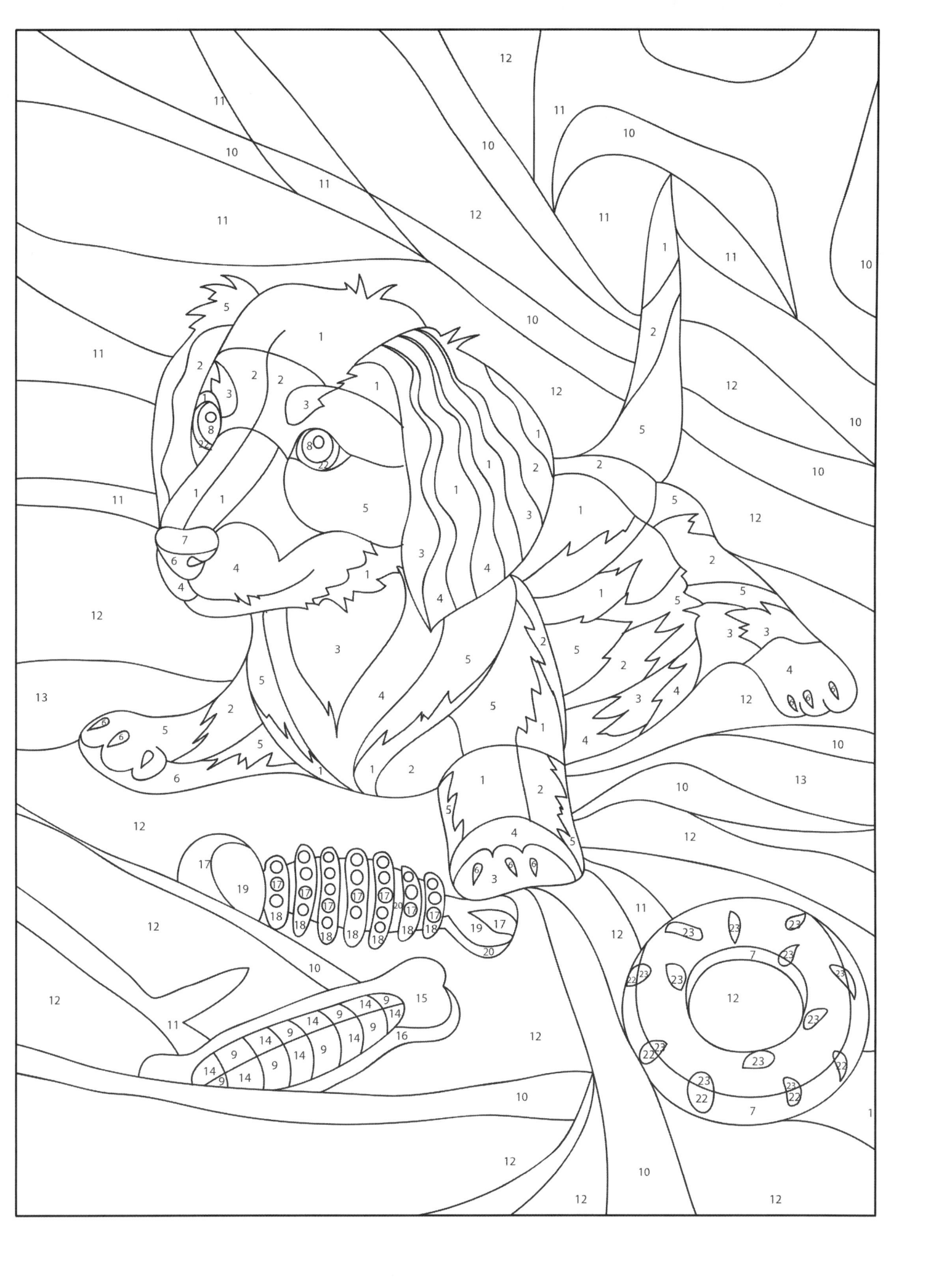

1. Dark Brown
2. Brown
3. Light Brown
4. Sand
5. Khaki
6. Dark Grey
7. Light Grey
8. Black
9. Light Pink
10. Pink
11. Magenta
12. Purple
13. Yellow
14. Gold
15. Orange
16. Red
17. Lime
18. Green
19. Light Green
20. Forrest Green
21. Blue Purple
22. Deep Blue
23. Sky Blue
24. Pale Blue

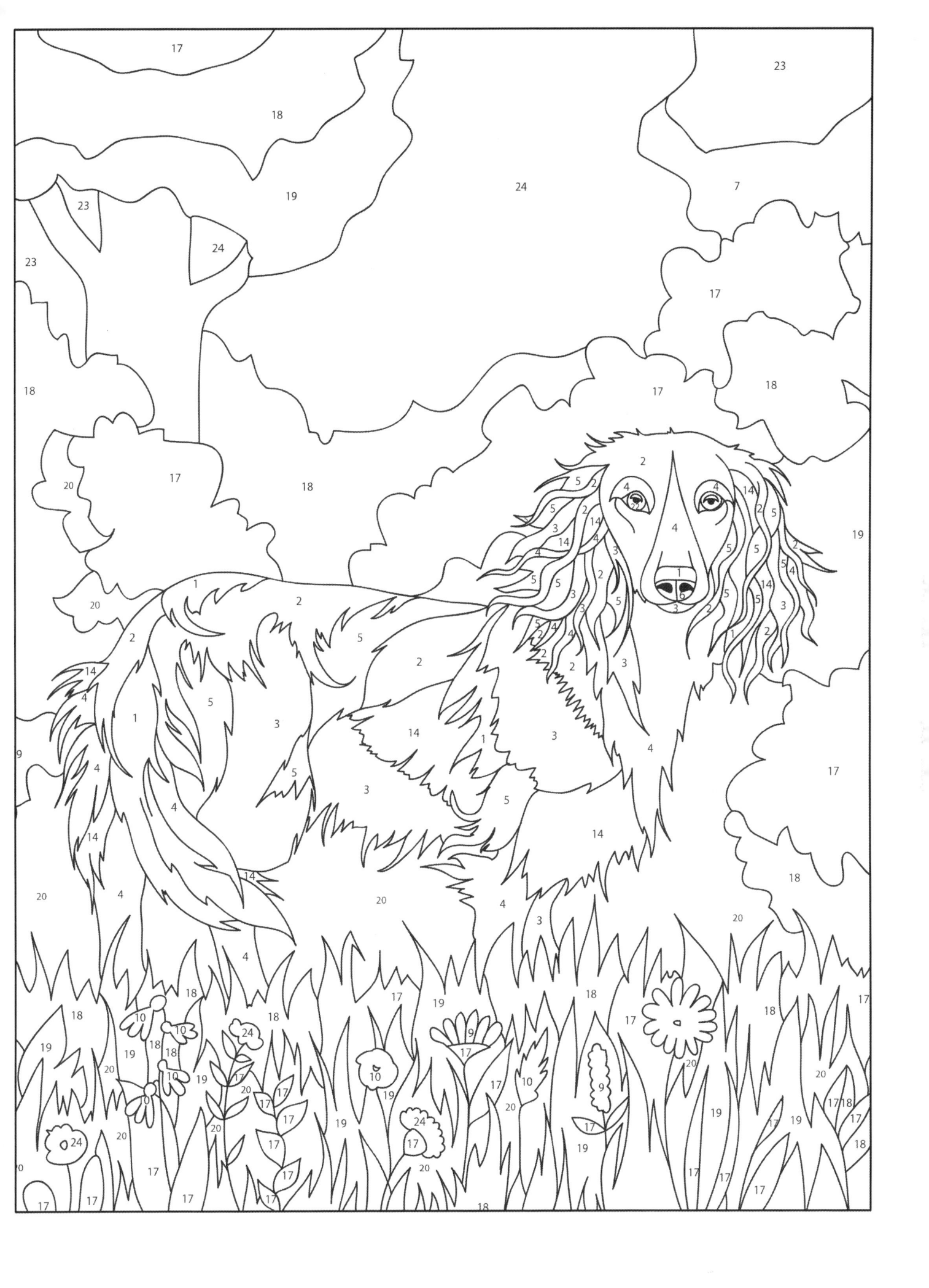

1. Dark Brown
2. Brown
3. Light Brown
4. Sand
5. Khaki
6. Dark Grey
7. Light Grey
8. Black
9. Light Pink
10. Pink
11. Magenta
12. Purple
13. Yellow
14. Gold
15. Orange
16. Red
17. Lime
18. Green
19. Light Green
20. Forrest Green
21. Blue Purple
22. Deep Blue
23. Sky Blue
24. Pale Blue

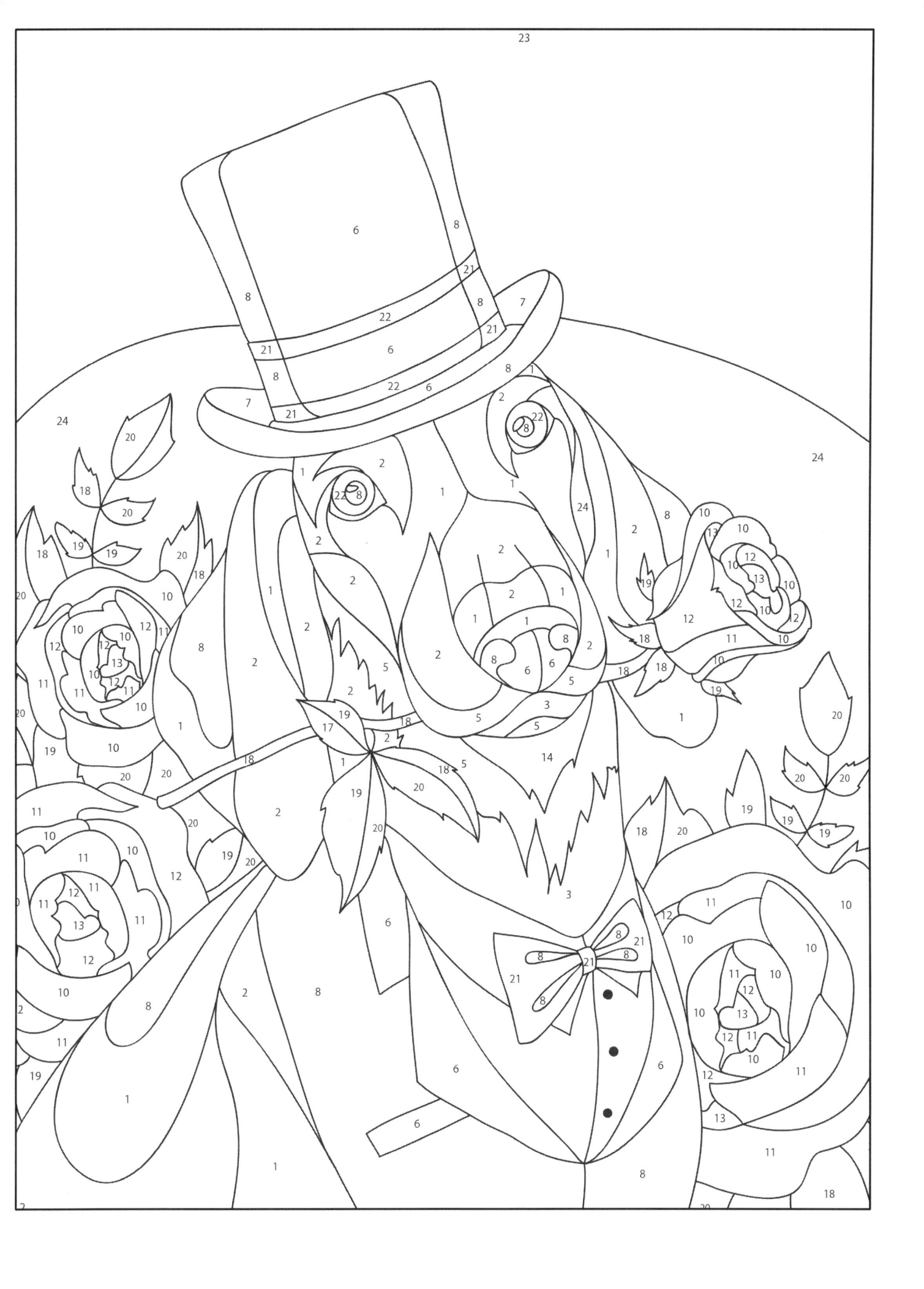

1. Dark Brown
2. Brown
3. Light Brown
4. Sand
5. Khaki
6. Dark Grey
7. Light Grey
8. Black
9. Light Pink
10. Pink
11. Magenta
12. Purple
13. Yellow
14. Gold
15. Orange
16. Red
17. Lime
18. Green
19. Light Green
20. Forrest Green
21. Blue Purple
22. Deep Blue
23. Sky Blue
24. Pale Blue

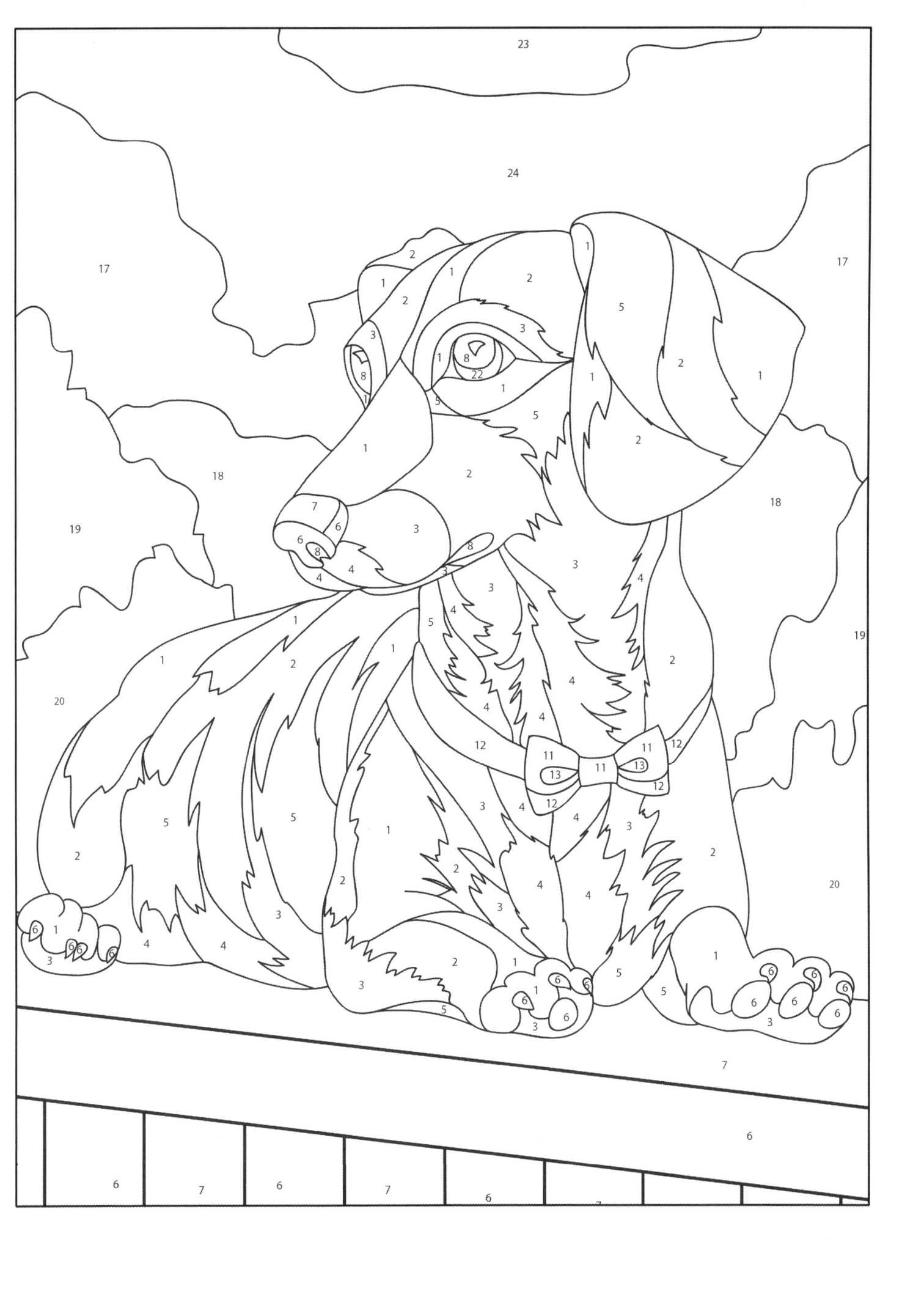

1. Dark Brown
2. Brown
3. Light Brown
4. Sand
5. Khaki
6. Dark Grey
7. Light Grey
8. Black
9. Light Pink
10. Pink
11. Magenta
12. Purple
13. Yellow
14. Gold
15. Orange
16. Red
17. Lime
18. Green
19. Light Green
20. Forrest Green
21. Blue Purple
22. Deep Blue
23. Sky Blue
24. Pale Blue

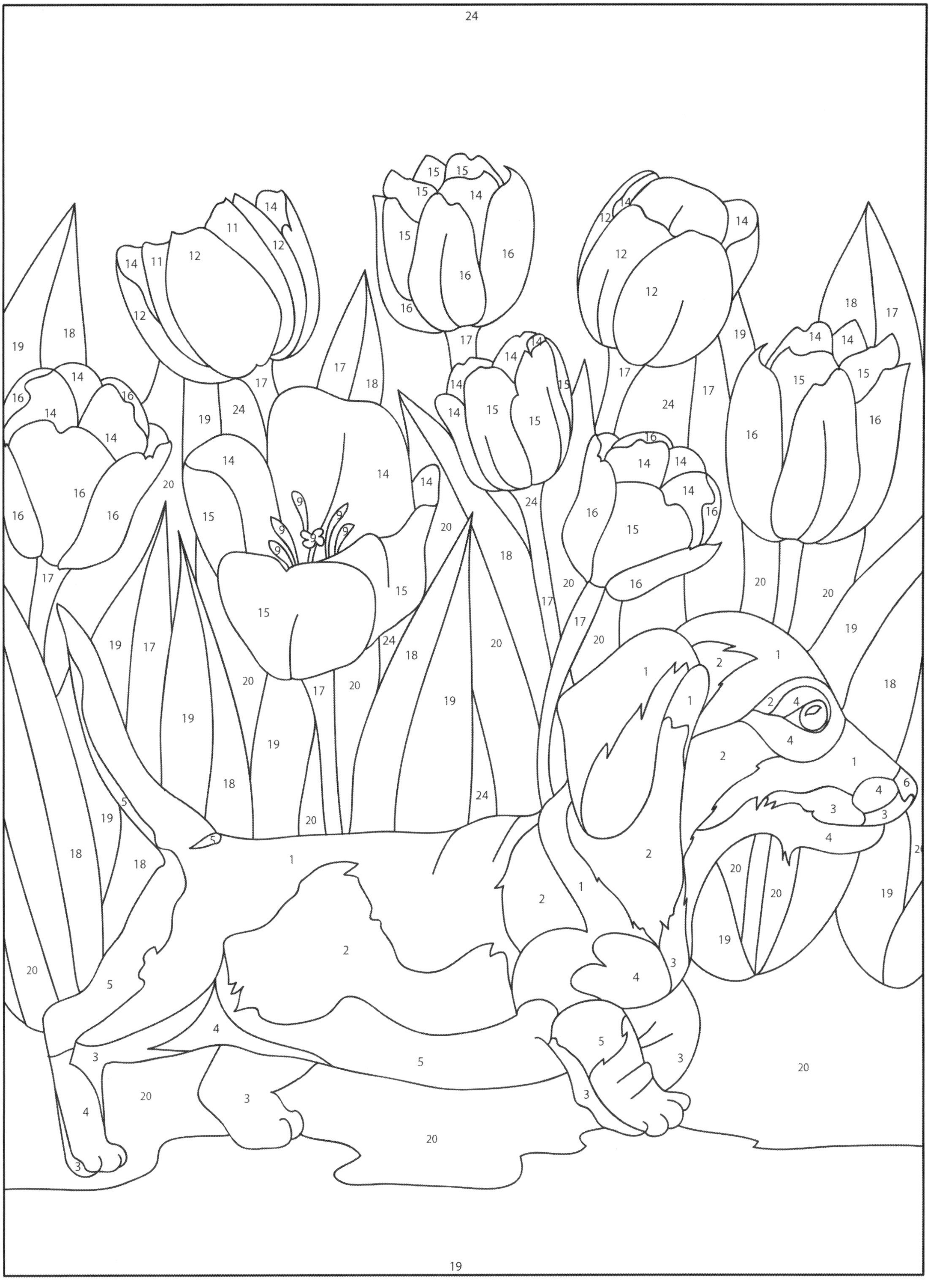

1. Dark Brown
2. Brown
3. Light Brown
4. Sand
5. Khaki
6. Dark Grey
7. Light Grey
8. Black
9. Light Pink
10. Pink
11. Magenta
12. Purple
13. Yellow
14. Gold
15. Orange
16. Red
17. Lime
18. Green
19. Light Green
20. Forrest Green
21. Blue Purple
22. Deep Blue
23. Sky Blue
24. Pale Blue

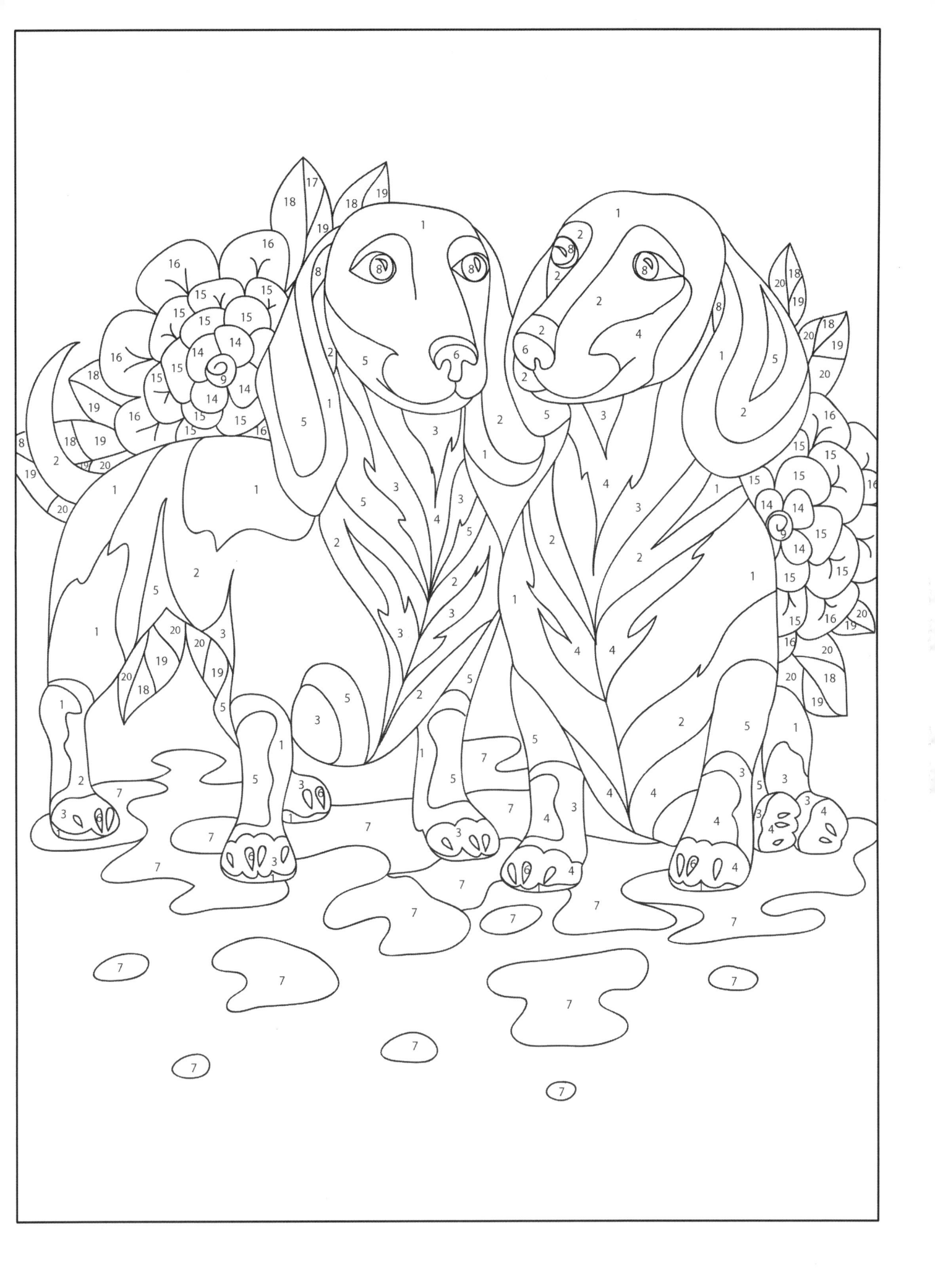

1. Dark Brown
2. Brown
3. Light Brown
4. Sand
5. Khaki
6. Dark Grey
7. Light Grey
8. Black
9. Light Pink
10. Pink
11. Magenta
12. Purple
13. Yellow
14. Gold
15. Orange
16. Red
17. Lime
18. Green
19. Light Green
20. Forrest Green
21. Blue Purple
22. Deep Blue
23. Sky Blue
24. Pale Blue

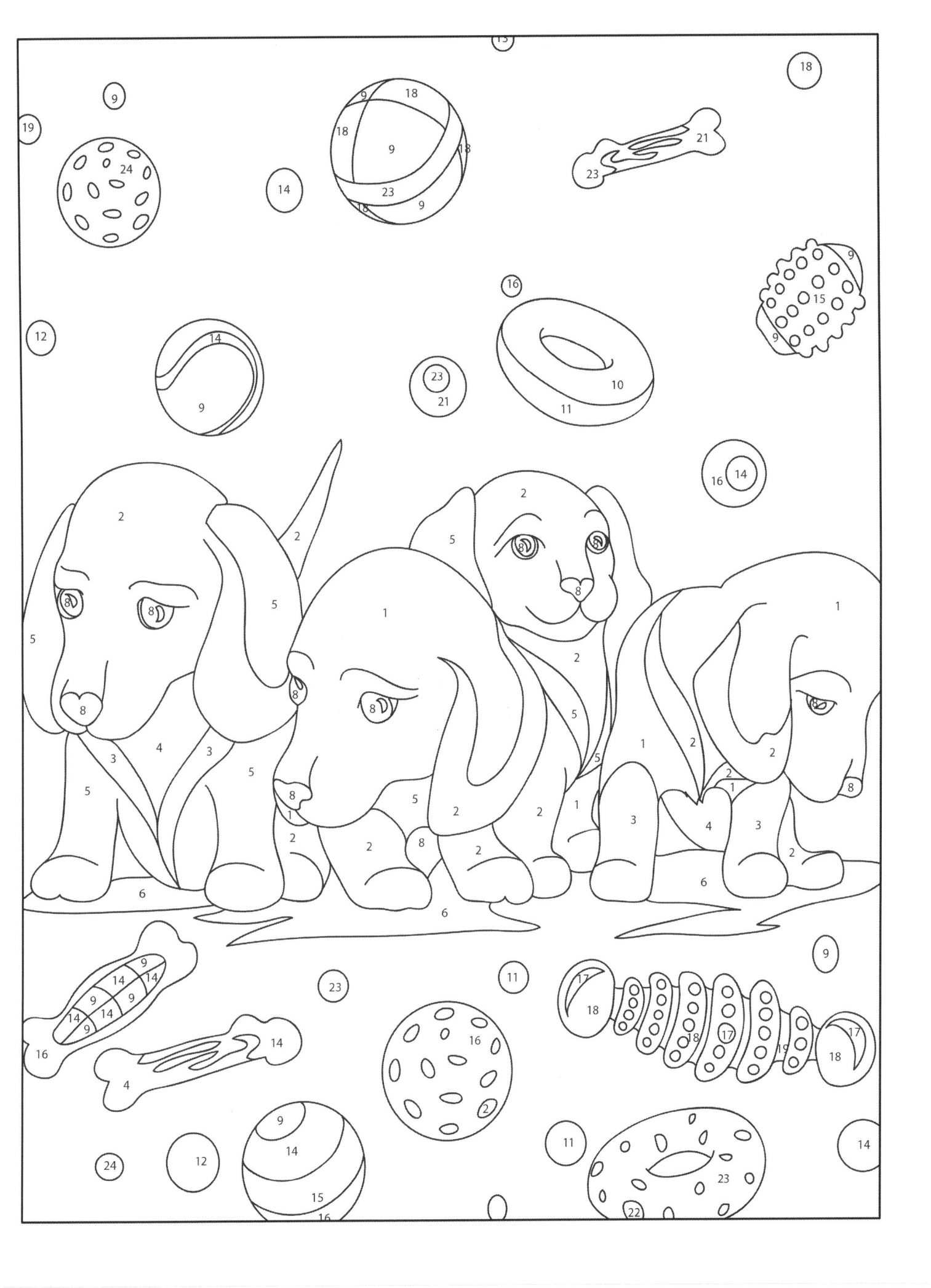

1. Dark Brown
2. Brown
3. Light Brown
4. Sand
5. Khaki
6. Dark Grey
7. Light Grey
8. Black
9. Light Pink
10. Pink
11. Magenta
12. Purple
13. Yellow
14. Gold
15. Orange
16. Red
17. Lime
18. Green
19. Light Green
20. Forrest Green
21. Blue Purple
22. Deep Blue
23. Sky Blue
24. Pale Blue

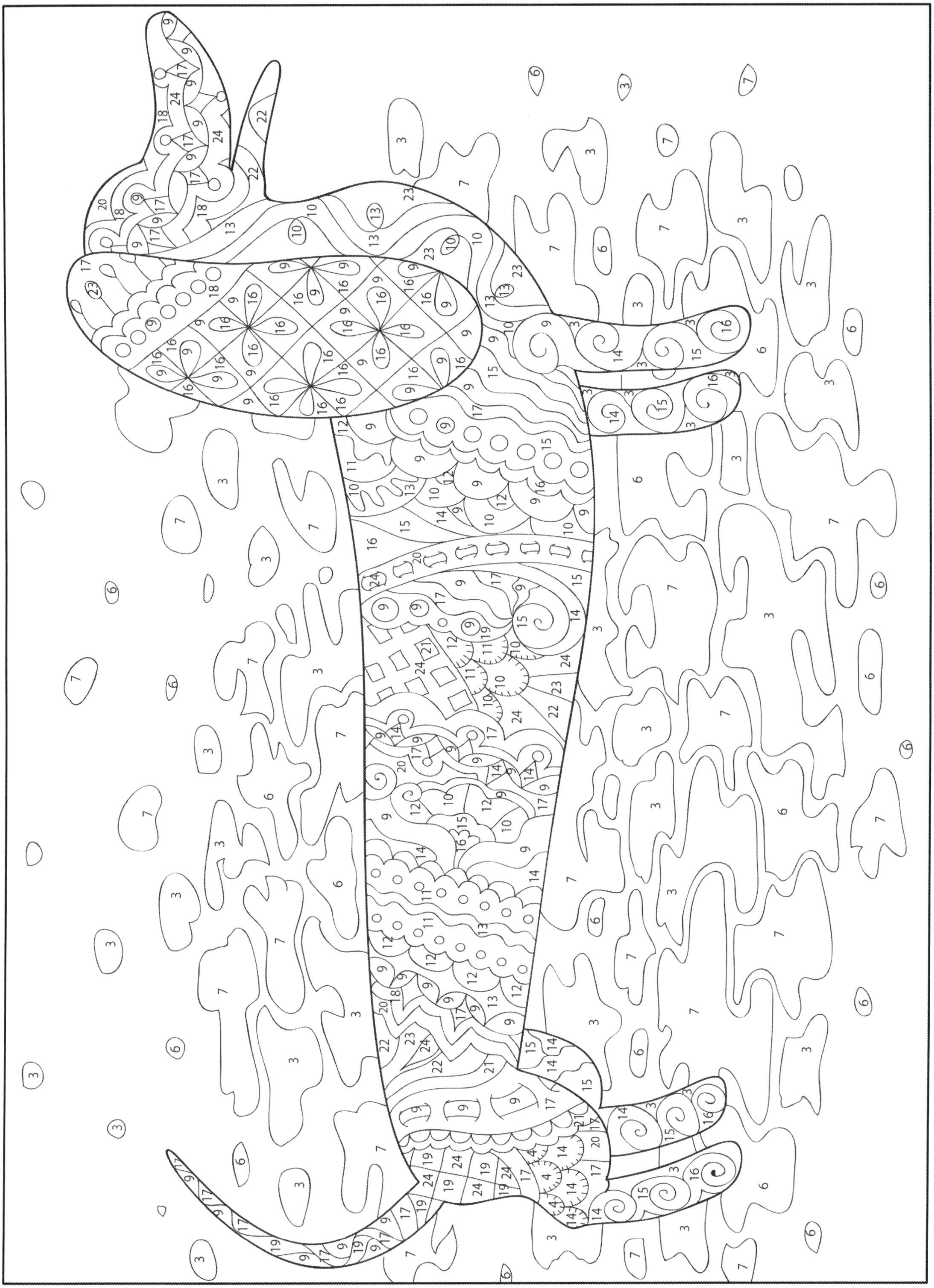

1. Dark Brown
2. Brown
3. Light Brown
4. Sand
5. Khaki
6. Dark Grey
7. Light Grey
8. Black
9. Light Pink
10. Pink
11. Magenta
12. Purple
13. Yellow
14. Gold
15. Orange
16. Red
17. Lime
18. Green
19. Light Green
20. Forrest Green
21. Blue Purple
22. Deep Blue
23. Sky Blue
24. Pale Blue

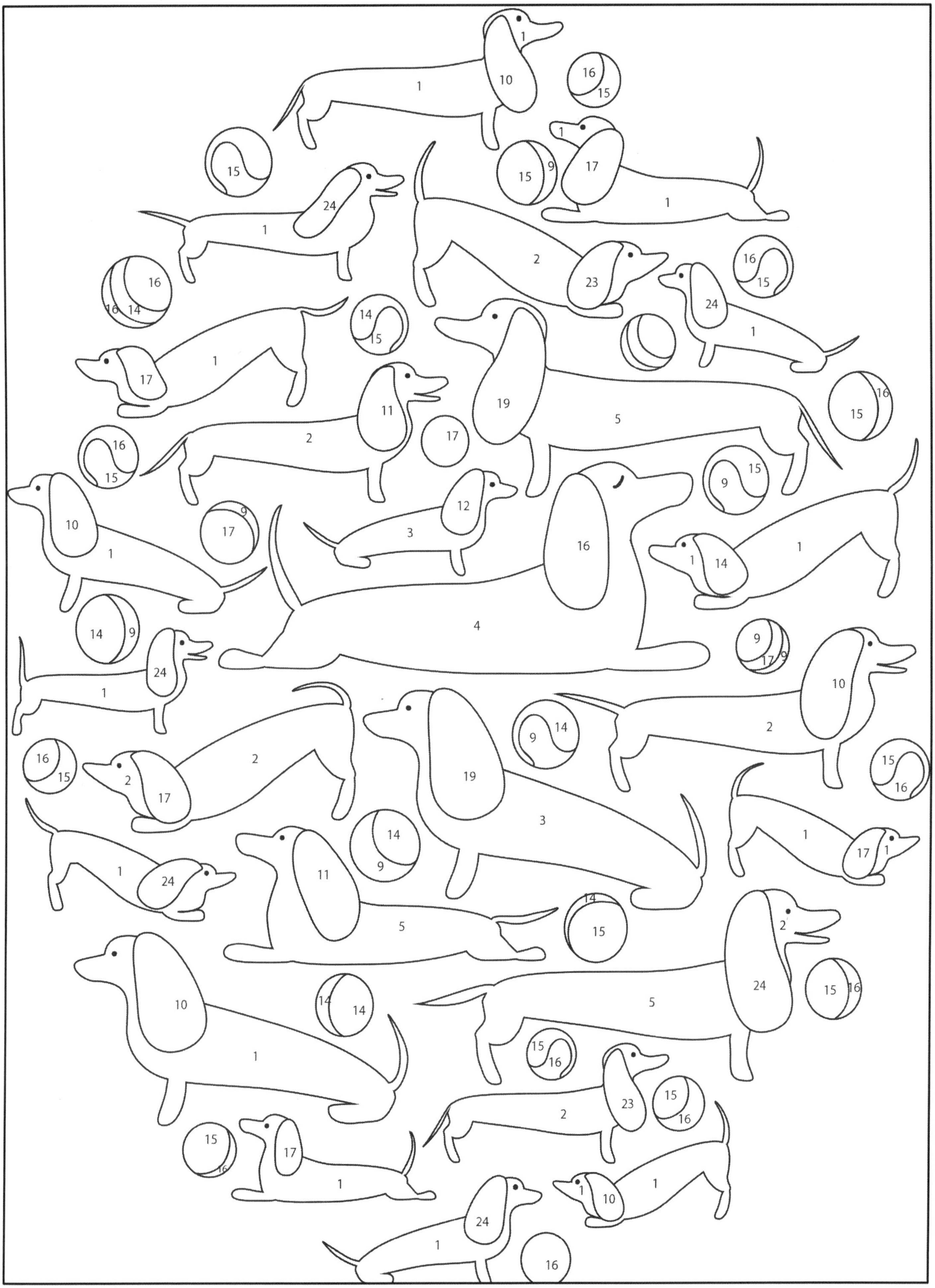

1. Dark Brown
2. Brown
3. Light Brown
4. Sand
5. Khaki
6. Dark Grey
7. Light Grey
8. Black
9. Light Pink
10. Pink
11. Magenta
12. Purple
13. Yellow
14. Gold
15. Orange
16. Red
17. Lime
18. Green
19. Light Green
20. Forrest Green
21. Blue Purple
22. Deep Blue
23. Sky Blue
24. Pale Blue

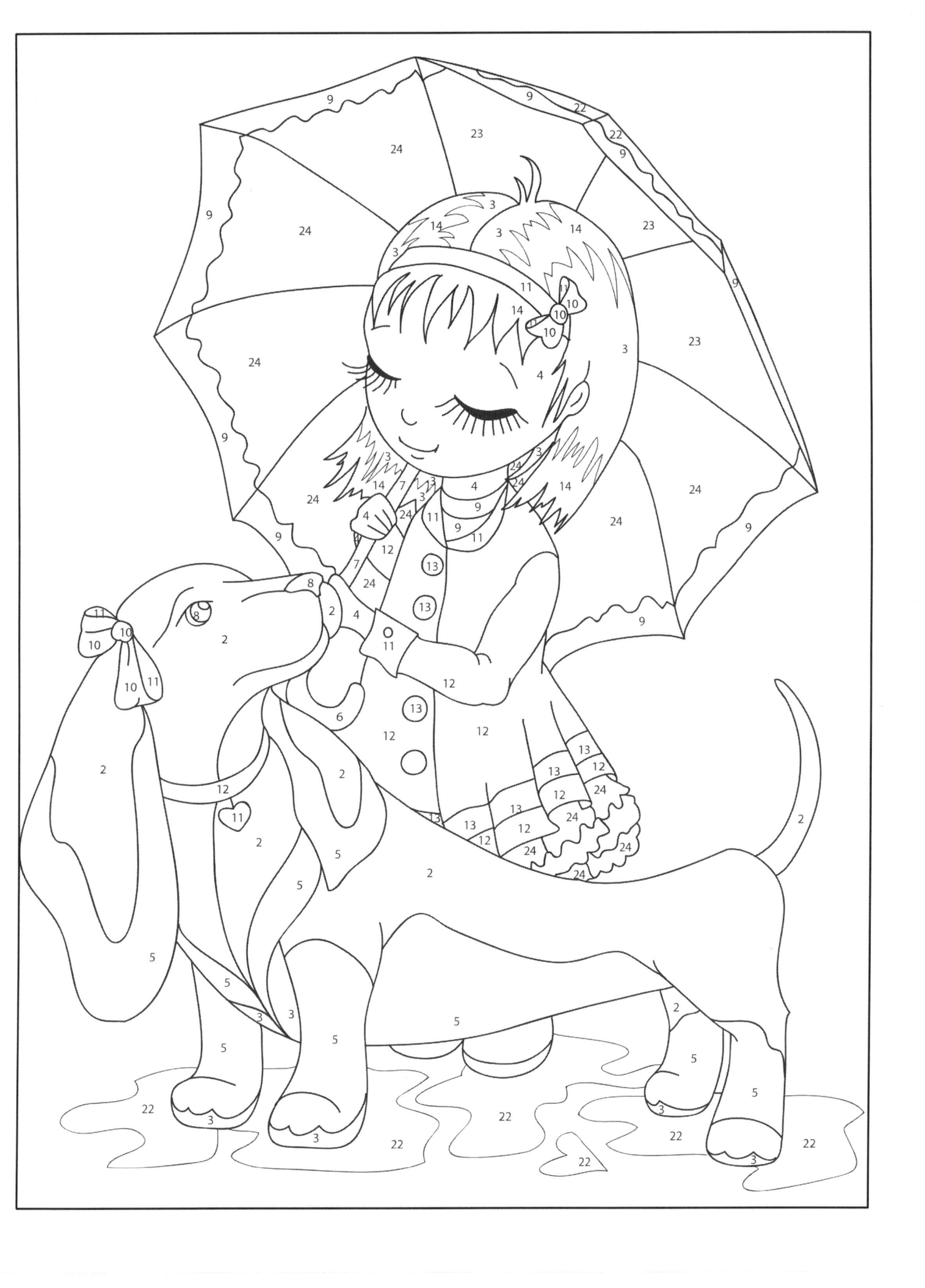

1. Dark Brown
2. Brown
3. Light Brown
4. Sand
5. Khaki
6. Dark Grey
7. Light Grey
8. Black
9. Light Pink
10. Pink
11. Magenta
12. Purple
13. Yellow
14. Gold
15. Orange
16. Red
17. Lime
18. Green
19. Light Green
20. Forrest Green
21. Blue Purple
22. Deep Blue
23. Sky Blue
24. Pale Blue

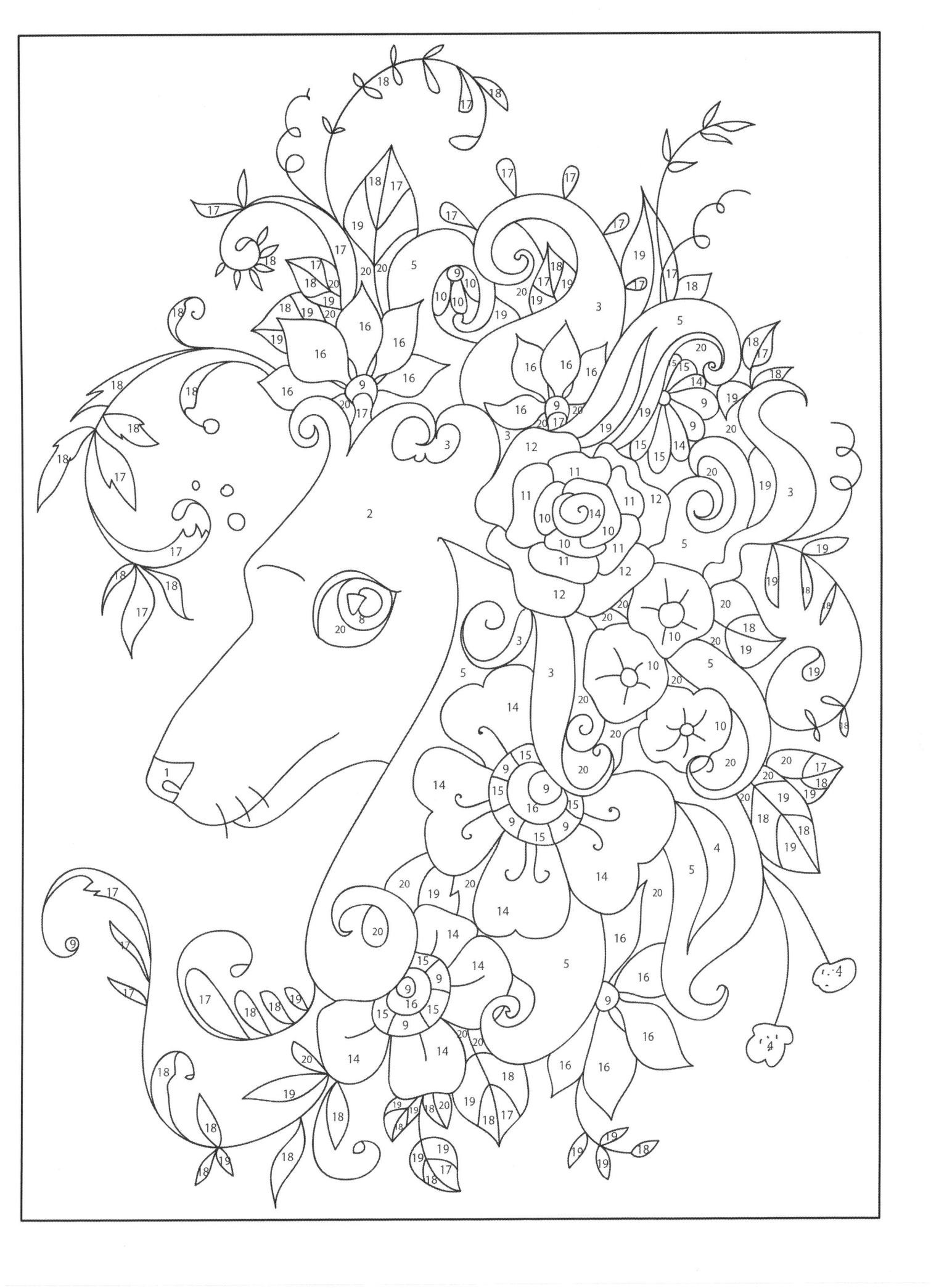

1. Dark Brown
2. Brown
3. Light Brown
4. Sand
5. Khaki
6. Dark Grey
7. Light Grey
8. Black
9. Light Pink
10. Pink
11. Magenta
12. Purple
13. Yellow
14. Gold
15. Orange
16. Red
17. Lime
18. Green
19. Light Green
20. Forrest Green
21. Blue Purple
22. Deep Blue
23. Sky Blue
24. Pale Blue

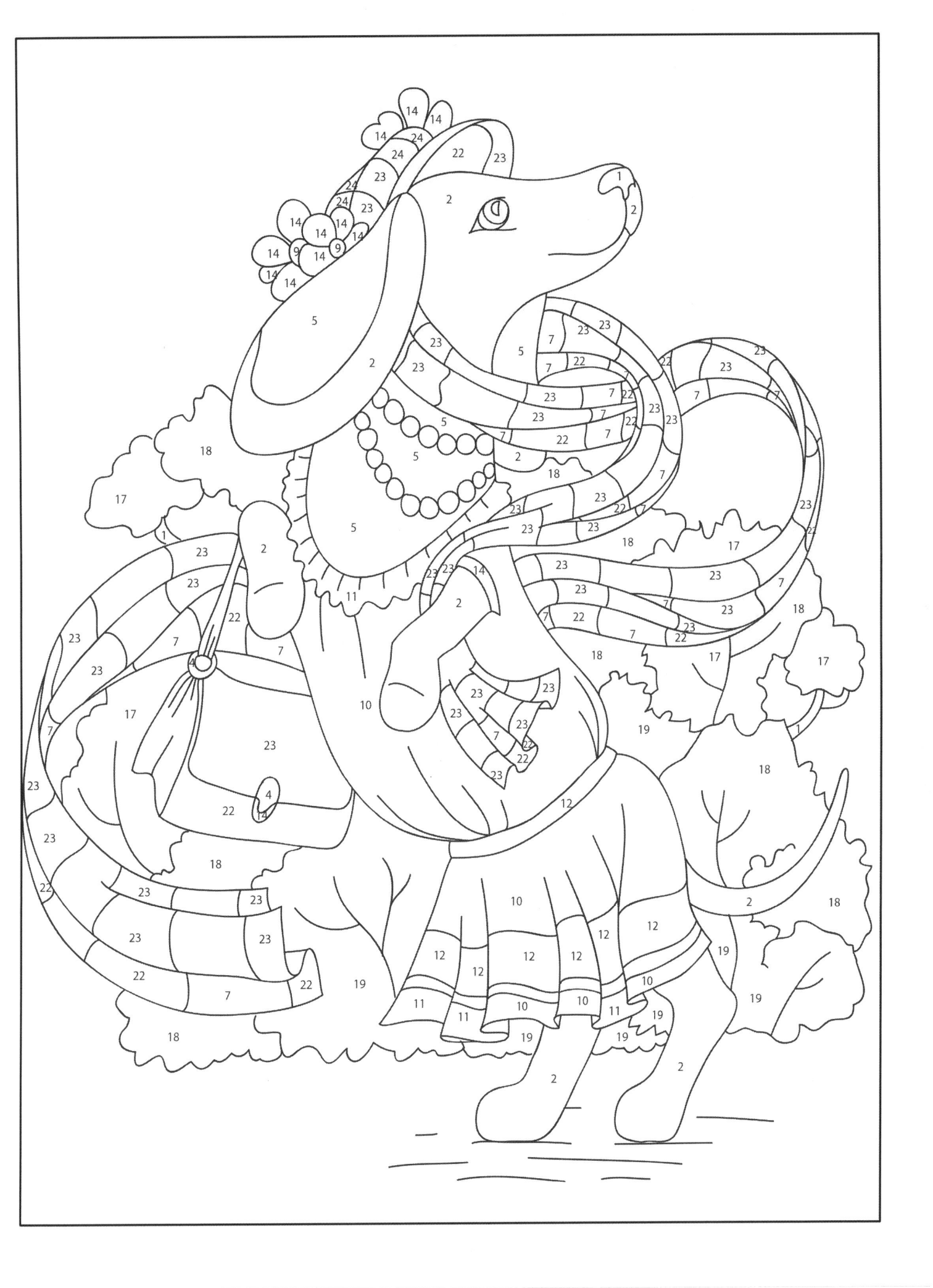

1. Dark Brown
2. Brown
3. Light Brown
4. Sand
5. Khaki
6. Dark Grey
7. Light Grey
8. Black
9. Light Pink
10. Pink
11. Magenta
12. Purple
13. Yellow
14. Gold
15. Orange
16. Red
17. Lime
18. Green
19. Light Green
20. Forrest Green
21. Blue Purple
22. Deep Blue
23. Sky Blue
24. Pale Blue

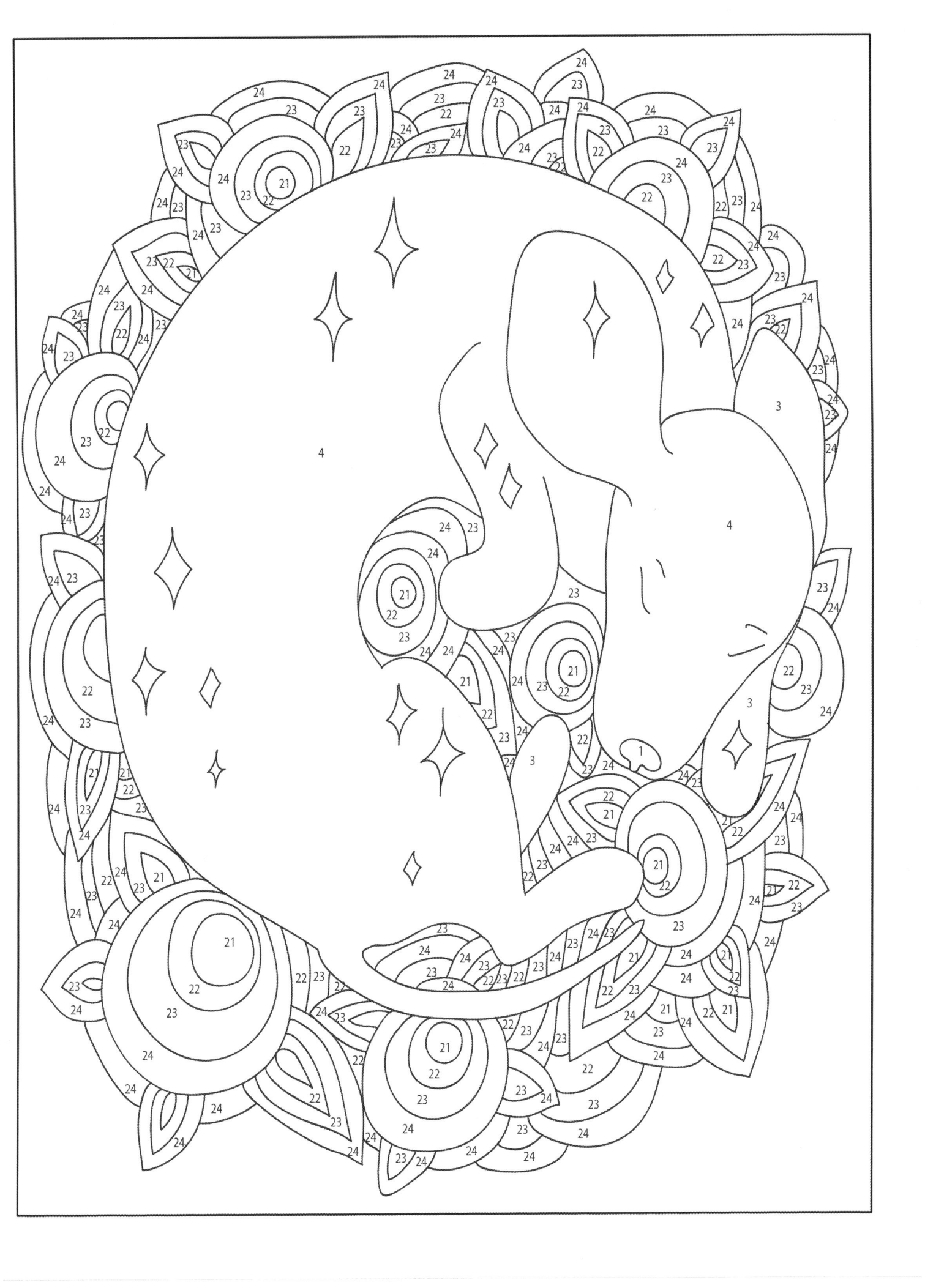

Thank you for supporting
ZenMaster Coloring Books

Your support means the world to us,
and we're thrilled to have you embark on this
creative journey with us.

Our small company strives to make a
BIG difference by helping those
who may be less fortunate.

This is why we proudly hire struggling
artists from around the world!

Our goal is to provide financial support to artists and
their families by enabling them to pursue their passions
and share their hard work and limitless talent with you!

Help support our hard working artists
by leaving a positive review on Amazon!

And follow us on Facebook for updates and
FREE COLORING PAGES!
https://www.facebook.com/zenmastercoloringbooks/

Check out more of our books at:
amazon.com/author/zenmastercoloringbooks

Free Bonus Page!
from:

Large Print Adult Coloring Book of
Kittens and Cats

https://www.amazon.com/dp/1983684775

Also available in color by numbers!!
https://www.amazon.com/dp/1983687626

And 5x8" Travel Size
https://www.amazon.com/dp/1727552121

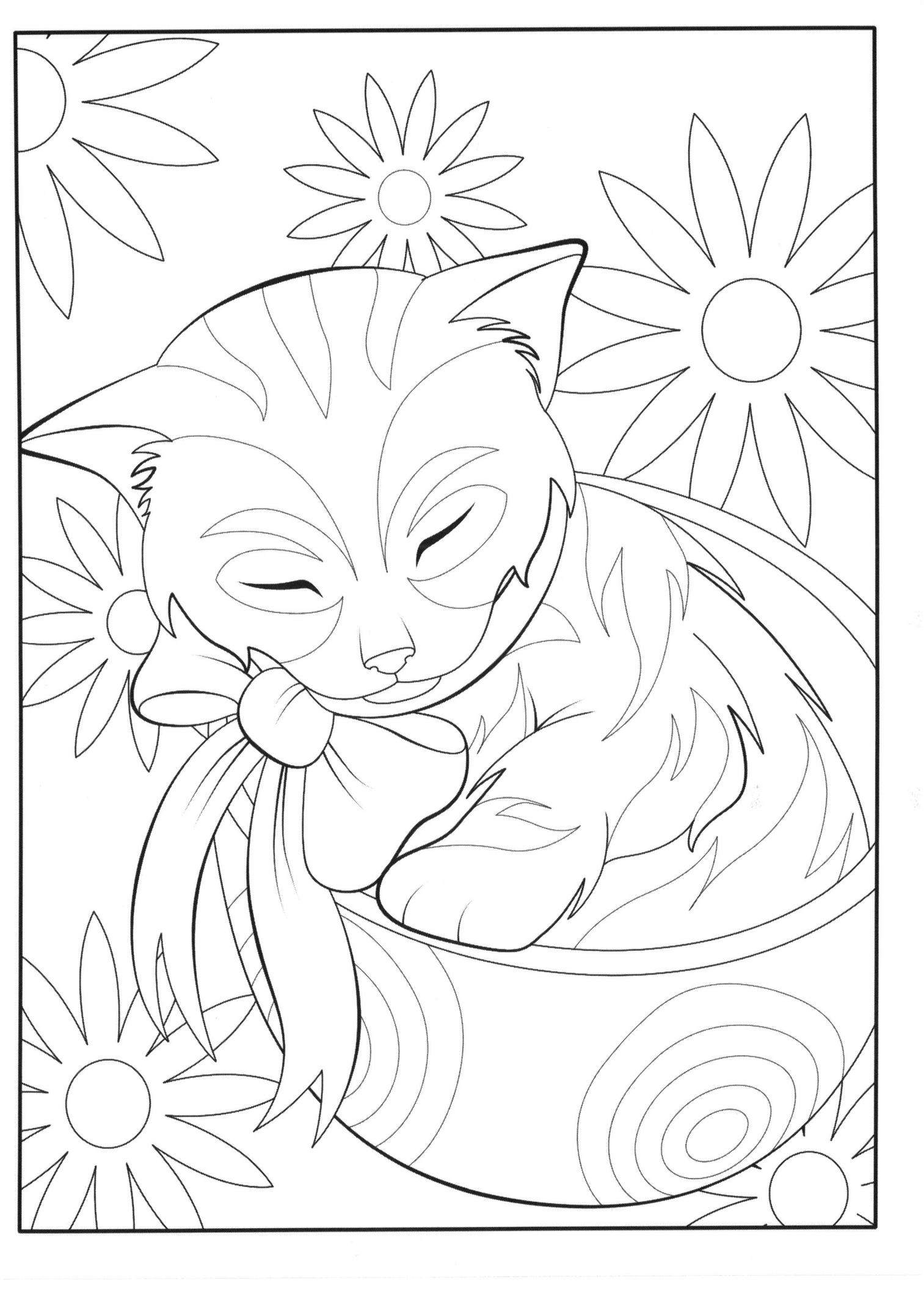

Free Bonus Page!
from:

Large Print Adult Coloring Book of
Mermaids

https://www.amazon.com/dp/1726089274

Also available in color by numbers!!
https://www.amazon.com/dp/1726069745

And 5x8" Travel Size
https://www.amazon.com/dp/1726398315

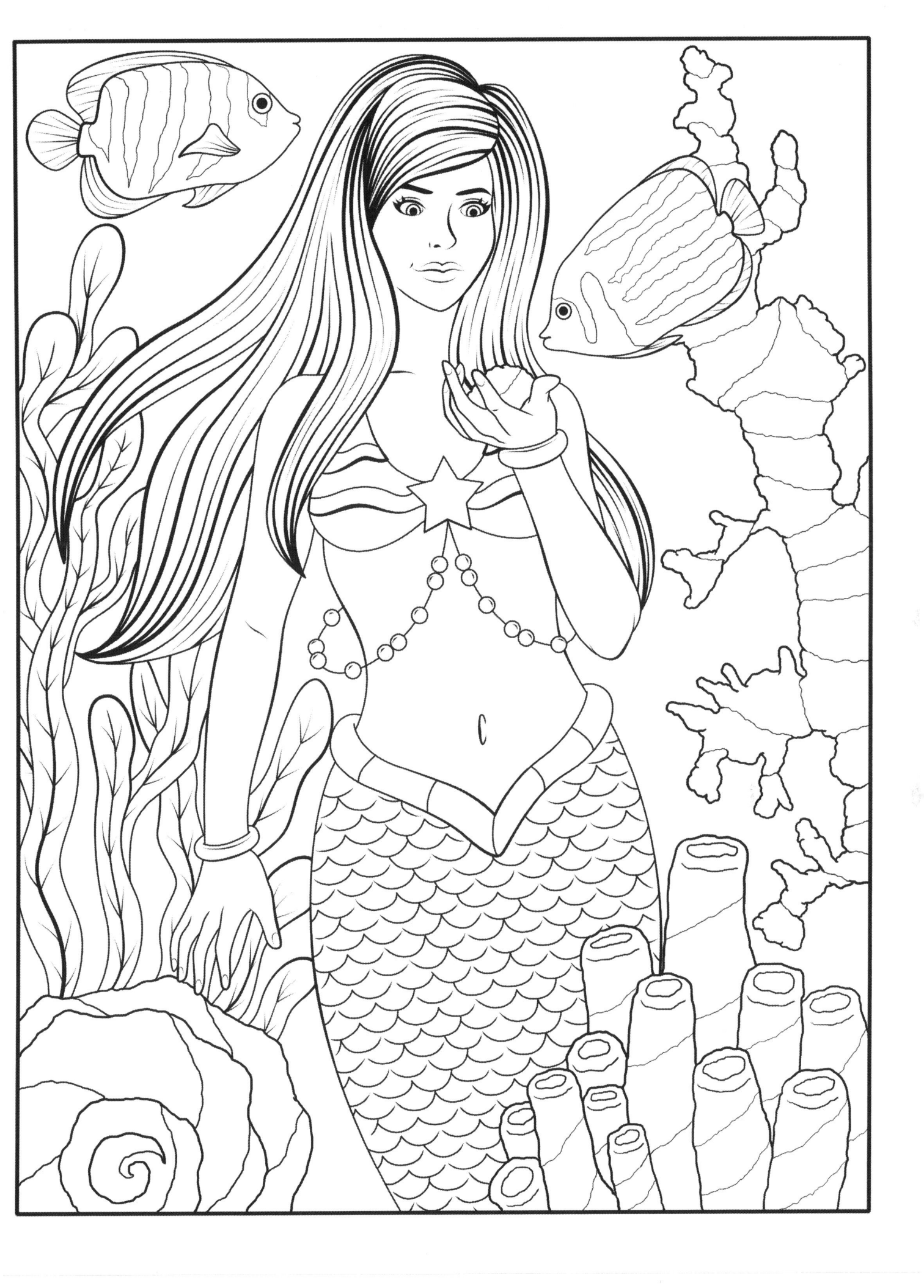

Free Bonus Page!
from:

Butterflies and Gardens
Large Pring Coloring Book for Adults

https://www.amazon.com/dp/1977882978

Also available in color by numbers!!
https://www.amazon.com/dp/1977932398

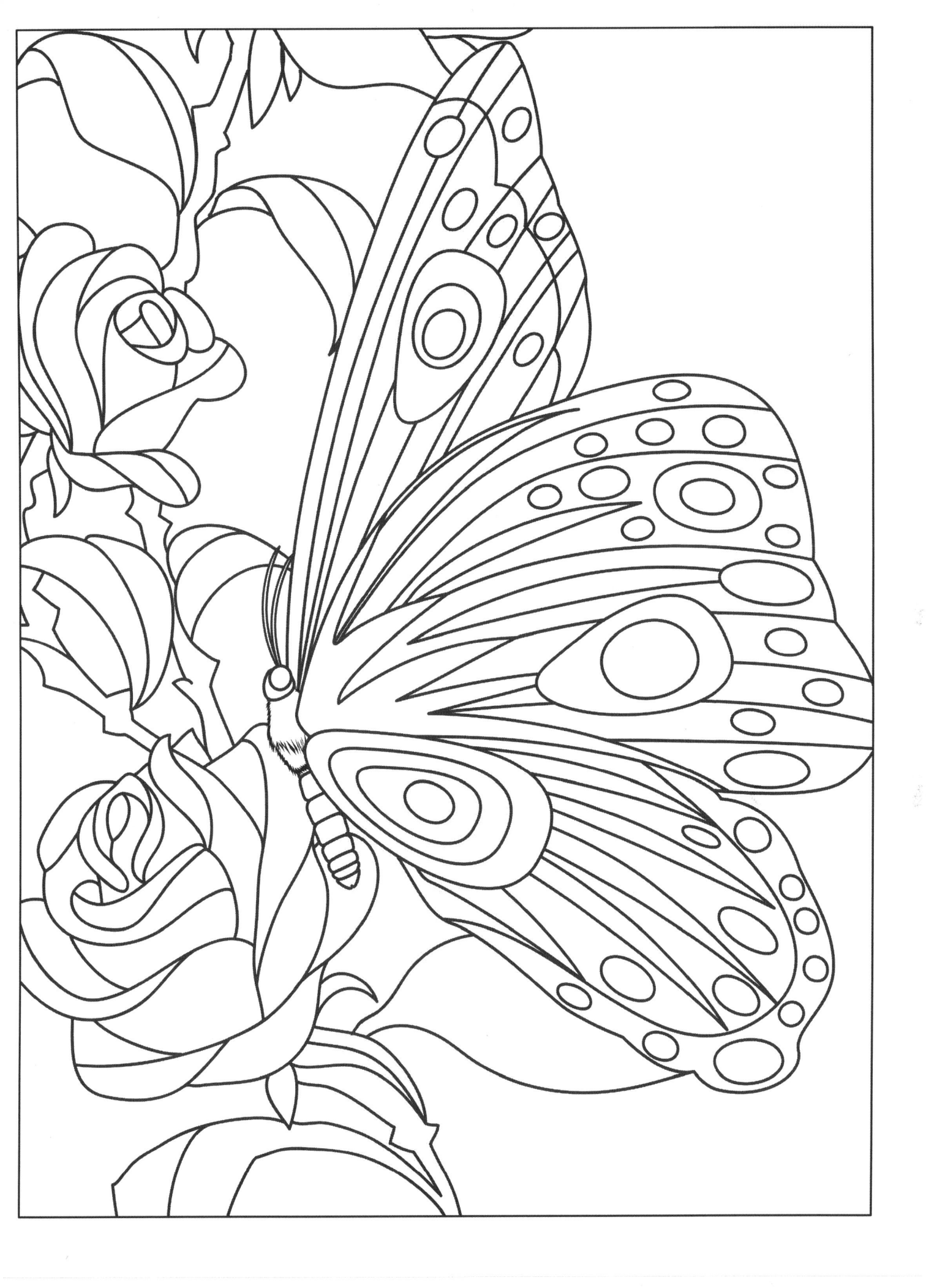

Free Bonus Page!
from:

Large Print Simple and Easy
Horses

https://www.amazon.com/dp/1977777775

Also available in color by numbers!!
https://www.amazon.com/dp/1977877176

And 5x8" Travel Size
https://www.amazon.com/dp/1727133811

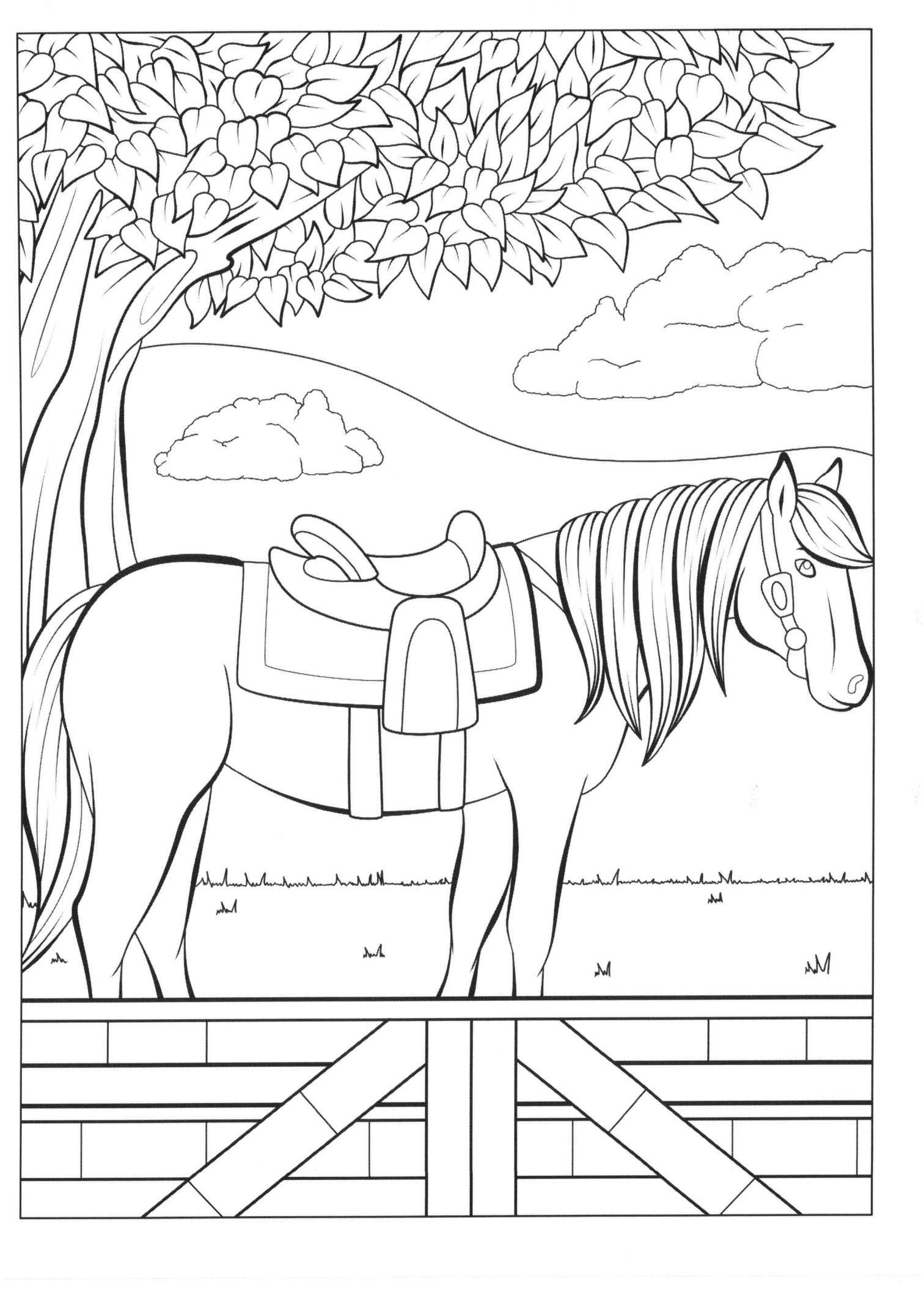

Free Bonus Page!
from:

Large Print Simple and Easy
Mandalas

https://www.amazon.com/dp/198151290x

Also available in color by numbers!!
https://amzn.com/dp/198207616x

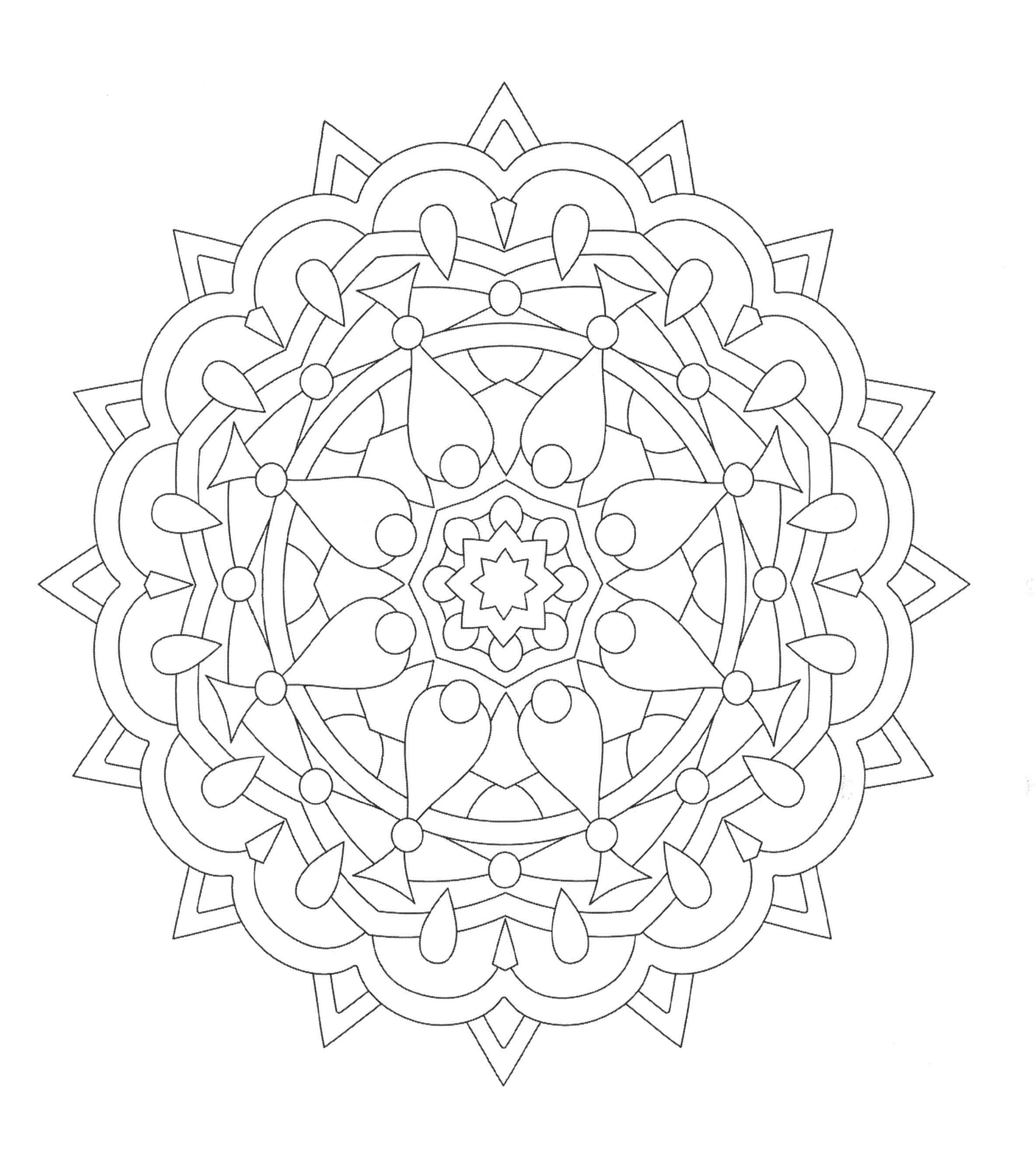

Free Bonus Page!
from:

Adult Coloring Book of
Sweets and Treats

https://www.amazon.com/dp/1795668881

Also available in color by numbers!!
https://www.amazon.com/dp/1795670983

And 5x8" Travel Size
https://www.amazon.com/dp/1796511447

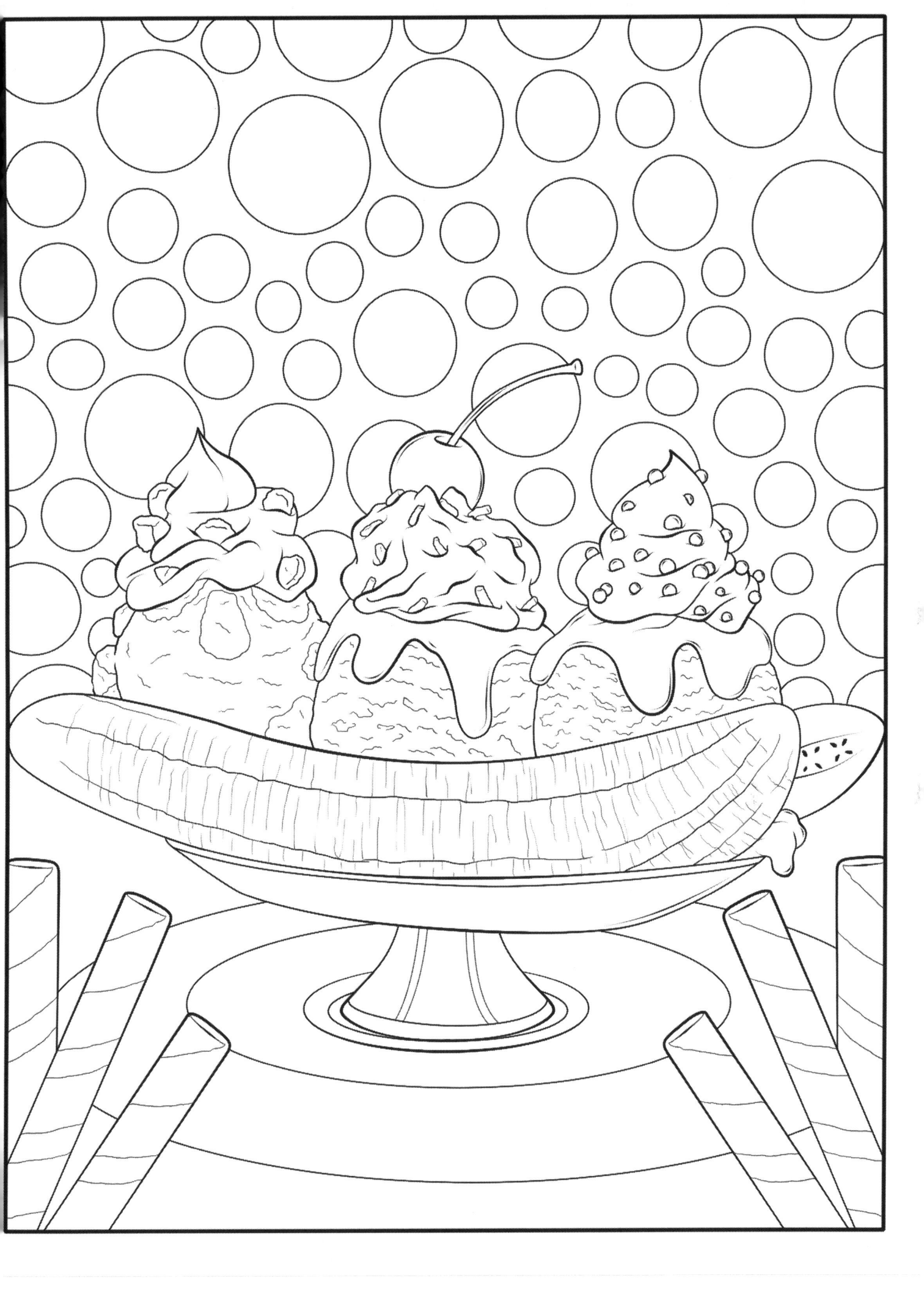

Free Bonus Page! from:

Zen Coloring Notebook

https://www.amazon.com/dp/1535457015

Available in 9 different colors!

Also available in 5x8" journal size

https://www.amazon.com/dp/1535540591

Made in the USA
Columbia, SC
10 June 2025